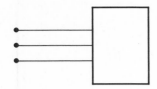

STATES, REGULATION AND
THE MEDICAL PROFESSION

SO-AZP-922

LAW AND POLITICAL CHANGE

Series Editors: Cosmo Graham and Professor Norman Lewis,
Centre for Socio-legal Studies, University of Sheffield

Forthcoming titles in the series:

J. Scott Davidson: *Human Rights*
Norman Lewis and Patrick Birkinshaw: *When Citizens Complain*

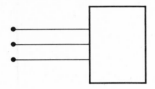

STATES, REGULATION AND THE MEDICAL PROFESSION

Michael Moran and Bruce Wood

OPEN UNIVERSITY PRESS
Buckingham • Philadelphia

Open University Press
Celtic Court
22 Ballmoor
Buckingham
MK18 1XW

and
1900 Frost Road, Suite 101
Bristol, PA 19007, USA

First Published 1993

Copyright © Michael Moran and Bruce Wood 1993

All rights reserved. No part of this publication may be
reproduced, stored in a retrieval system or transmitted
in any form or by any means, without written permission
from the publisher.

A catalogue record of this book is available
from the British Library

Library of Congress Cataloging-in-Publication Data
Moran, Michael.
    States, regulation and the medical profession/Michael Moran and
Bruce Wood.
        p.   cm.
    Includes bibliographical references and index.
    ISBN 0–335–15749–1 (hard). — ISBN 0–335–15748–3 (pbk.)
    1. Medical policy—United States.   2. Medical policy—Great
Britain.   3. Medical policy—Germany.   4. Medical policy—Cross-
cultural studies.   I. Wood, Bruce.   II. Title.
RA393.M627   1992
362.1—dc20   92–23833
                                                                              CIP

Typeset by Colset Private Limited, Singapore
Printed in Great Britain by Biddles Ltd, Guildford and Kings Lynn

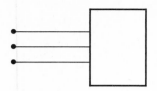

CONTENTS

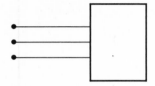

PREFACE

THE PURPOSE OF THIS BOOK

States, Regulation and the Medical Profession is written for students – both of medicine and of social science. It introduces a subject which is of vital concern to doctors and to their patients: just how, and to what extent, is the occupation of medicine regulated, and what role does the state play in that regulation?

At first sight the involvement of states in the politics of health care is considerable. In most developed countries issues about health are high on the domestic political agenda. This is not surprising, for two reasons. First, everyone wants to enjoy good health and to live for as long as possible, and so access to good health care is a highly valued possession. Second, the provision of health care is a costly exercise, and someone has to pay the bill.

Health and health care are major political issues whether or not the state takes responsibility for ensuring access, providing facilities or paying the bill. In the UK, for example, there is through the National Health Service heavy government involvement in all three activities, whereas in the USA government plays a relatively minor role.

Whether or not the state provides or pays for health care, it is certain to be interested in the regulation of doctors. Medicine is so central to modern society that doctors have emerged as perhaps the key profession. The extent to which they are regulated, and the nature of any governmental involvement in that regulation, is thus a matter of widespread interest and concern.

Scope and structure

This book is a comparative study of three important industrialized, Western nations. Our premise is that while it is always valuable for students to learn about the country in which they happen to live or study, comparisons across borders add enormously to our understanding of what we can so easily assume is 'the norm' everywhere. We thus address the extent to which arrangements in one country for the regulation of doctors resemble, or differ from, those found elsewhere.

The three countries we examine are the UK, the USA and Germany. We choose the UK because its health-care system is internationally important: it is widely considered to be the leading example of the model of a health-care system known as a 'national health service'. Germany, too, was chosen because it pioneered a different way of organizing health care. The German system, usually called the 'compulsory insurance model', has been widely imitated both on the continent of Europe and in Canada. But any account of Germany now has to be tentative. When we began this book our interest was in the Federal Republic of Germany, commonly known as West Germany. There also existed a smaller German state in the east, the German Democratic Republic, whose economy (and health-care service) were run almost entirely by government. That state collapsed in 1989, and in 1990 was incorporated into the Federal Republic. The intention is to dismantle the previous East German health-care system, replacing it with the system in the West. However, there is now a state of transition. Our account of Germany is largely based on arrangements in the old 'West' Germany. These arrangements will undoubtedly be dominant in the new Germany. However, where parts of the old East German system are likely to survive, we describe them.

The UK and Germany were natural selections partly because of their size. Our third country, the US, is, of course, even larger. By most measures it is the biggest health-care system in the world. In addition, its organization remains unique: it is the one nation in the rich, 'developed' world where market forces remain important in the direct relationship between doctor (or physician) and patient.

In Chapter 1 the American 'pluralist' or 'market-based' health-care system will be briefly outlined and described, as will the German and UK models. The opening chapter also introduces doctors in their several guises – as medical practitioners, as politicians, and as economic actors. Chapter 2 is designed to give the reader the 'academic background' – to sketch the main issues raised in the study of how the medical profession is regulated. Chapter 3 looks at how regulation developed historically in each state. Against this historical background, Chapter 4 describes and compares the modern institutions of regulation. This chapter is designed to provide the 'bare bones' of regulation. Chapter 5 has the purpose of showing how the institutions work to produce policy. Chapter 6 examines the impact of all this activity on key groups such as patients, and on doctors themselves. Finally, Chapter 7 examines how far doctors are losing control over the regulation of their profession. Throughout the emphasis is on the relations between governments and doctors, and the regulation of the profession collectively. Relations between individual patients and their doctors, including details of the processes by which complaints are handled, lie largely outside the scope of our study.

Sources

This is a student text, not a monograph reporting original research. This influences our citation of sources. We have kept citation in the text to a minimum. Each chapter concludes with a note on sources, which also acts as a guide to further reading.

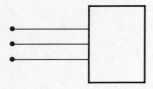

ACKNOWLEDGEMENTS

This book is the outcome of a major change of research direction for both of us. Our thanks go to the University of Manchester for the provision of an initial research award (and to Elizabeth Alexander, who made good use of that award in providing us with an initial bibliography); and for the granting of leave of absence to enable Bruce Wood to spend a semester studying in the USA. We are also grateful to the German Academic Exchange Service for funding Michael Moran to undertake research in Germany and to the series editors for their helpful comments on an earlier draft. Finally, Miss Marilyn Dunn performed heroics as interpreter-in-chief of our handwriting and as our personal wordprocessor.

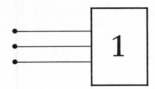

DOCTORS, STATES AND HEALTH CARE

DOCTORS

Healers. Scientists. Professionals. Entrepreneurs. Politicians. These five nouns have all been used (along with several other terms) to describe doctors. Taken collectively they convey, quite correctly, the notion that doctors, as individuals, provide valuable services to the sick and that, as a group, they are so powerful and significant that the modern state cannot ignore them and will have to deal with them. Taken individually, the five descriptions reflect the wide range of behavioural characteristics of doctors.

The doctor as a healer is almost god-like. The traditional one-to-one relationship between doctor and patient remains the cornerstone of medical ethics. The term healer, with its overtones of faith healing, reflects fairly the lack of absolute certainty in diagnosis and in treatment, and the fact that until not much more than a century ago, there were few effective treatments available. The traditional doctor gives hope and brings comfort; medicine is an art supported by a rapidly growing but imprecise technology. Doctors are called; medicine is a vocation.

The solo practitioner enjoying a direct personal relationship with the patient remains alive and well today. Among other places he is to be found in UK general practice and US family practice, still taking care in the more rural areas of all but the very specialized health needs of the population. But increasingly, the doctor is both part of a team and dependent on modern scientific discoveries. The team is sometimes made up of other doctors. A group of primary care doctors may work out of a single set of offices. In hospitals the surgeon works alongside the anaesthetist and in partnership with the radiologist and pathologist, reflecting the increased specialization of medicine. And the team sometimes includes other health professionals. To some extent diagnosis and, more especially, treatment is jointly determined and effected through the assistance of physiotherapists and other therapists, psychologists, technicians and, of course, nurses.

This growth of teamwork has paralleled the development of the doctor as scientist. To the stethoscope has been added the body scanner. To herbal remedies (which can often work) and folk remedies have been added the modern drugs manufactured by the pharmaceutical industry in the scientific laboratory. Doctors need to be aware of, if not have access to, an enormous range of new technologies which, collectively, have improved diagnosis and enabled new forms of treatment to be undertaken at a rate never before experienced. Medicine, still an art, has become a science. Doctors are thus, partly, scientists.

That doctors are professionals is a normal belief: indeed, most would bracket doctors and lawyers as *the* classic examples of what is normally meant by a 'profession'. Characteristics commonly are said to include an agreed ethical code, discipline rules, and control of entry and training standards. (The accuracy of this we examine in Chapter 2.) Institutionally, recognition by the public of professional (and social) status is reflected in the expectation that doctors will be members of the appropriate professional organization. In the UK, recognition is symbolically by the very head of state. Hence there are the Royal Colleges of Surgeons, of Physicians, of General Practitioners. To this has been added parliamentary recognition of the virtues of professional self-regulation, and legislation creating a General Medical Council to determine whether or not a 'doctor' should obtain registration. The USA and Germany, though not monarchies, also have a long history of legislative and executive recognition of medicine as a profession.

These first three descriptions – healer, scientist, professional – paint a picture of the doctor as almost saint-like, selflessly devoted to patients, to the community, and to self-betterment so as to use the latest knowledge and treatments. He or she stands above the petty daily rancour of 'normal' human life, offering help and hope to the suffering. Not surprisingly, opinion polls show doctors to be widely respected and their opinions to be widely believed (though as we will see later, this respect may be fading).

There is, however, another side to the coin and it is reflected in the final two descriptions of 'entrepreneur' and 'politician'. Doctors are businessmen, part of the real economic world, in need of money. Two centuries ago they sought wealthy patrons and offered solace and comfort in exchange for accommodation or honoraria. Today few doctors can rely on only a handful of patients (exceptions include the almost full-time personal physicians of the US President and the British monarch). The norm is to rely on small pieces of income from many people or many activities.

A doctor's income may be received per patient (regardless of the amount of treatment given), per item of treatment, or by way of a salary. The payer may be the patient, an insurance company, a hospital, or the government. Whatever the system (and the system varies markedly from country to country, as will be seen later in this chapter), the normal economic tensions between payers and providers of any service exist. The doctor provider naturally seeks a healthy income, while the payer equally naturally wishes to limit outgoings. Disputes are inevitable from time to time. Because payers are nowadays largely private or public organizations, rather than individual patients, such disputes have wide repercussions for both parties, for the state, and for health care. Even in the most 'market run' of health-care systems – the USA – government cannot avoid becoming involved in doctor–payer relationships.

And this last involvement emphasizes that doctors are politicians. Both individually and, more significantly, as a group they possess and use many political resources. These include their positive public image; their expertise, time and skill in making a case; the many officials they employ to run their associations; their access to payer groups and to government; and the powerful sanctions at their disposal (for example, refusal to cooperate with imposed reforms, even withdrawal of labour). Doctors form powerful groups, notably the national medical associations, which often act like trade unions to defend the self-interest of members.

The political power of doctors has three dimensions. First, the profession can positively intervene in public policy debates about health care, functioning as an influential lobbyist. Later in the chapter we will see how US and UK doctors have struck deals with government affecting medical practice and doctors' incomes. Second, doctors have the power to influence the kinds of decisions which reach the public agenda. Their well-known opposition in the USA to the introduction of any form of national health insurance or service is one reason why national health insurance has never been a serious policy option in the USA. Third, doctors have structural power stemming from their position as professional monopolizers of accepted medical knowledge: their views on disease and illness tend to dominate health policy because they are recognized by society as the experts in the field.

STATES AND DOCTORS

States are central to the working lives of doctors. Even in the USA, with easily the lowest level of state provision of health care in any developed nation, public expenditure on health still accounts for 43 per cent of the total spending on health care. But the importance of the state goes beyond public spending. All states have good economic reasons for seeking to regulate the health-care providers.

States have three major concerns to consider – the costs of health care, the quality of treatment, and access to care. Their overall objectives are to keep costs down while simultaneously ensuring high standards of quality and good access to care. Clearly these are potentially incompatible as improvements to quality and to access are likely to add to costs. In seeking to 'square the circle' governments have designed, or allowed to grow, very different overall health-care systems, as the next three sections of this chapter will illustrate.

THE USA: A PLURALIST HEALTH-CARE SYSTEM

There is no single health-care system in the USA. Rather, it is best described as 'pluralist': the state plays an important role, but so also do markets. Most Americans carry health insurance through their employment. The package of benefits for the employee is met largely by the employer (often 80 per cent or 90 per cent of the premium), and the employee can include dependants in the policy, but frequently by meeting most of their premium. The insurers are predominantly not-for-profit organizations (Blue Cross and Blue Shield) set up in the 1930s, and a range of private-sector mutual assurance companies or, increasingly, Health Maintenance Organizations (HMOs) or Preferred Provider Organizations (PPOs), both of which provide care at reduced premiums.

The old and the poor are covered under the federal Medicare and the 50 separate state Medicaid programmes which, along with the small directly provided services for armed forces Veterans and for Indians, account for over 40 per cent of all health-care spending (Medicare provides for some of the old; Medicaid provides for some of the poor). But there are gaps, and for two reasons as many as 37 million Americans (or more than one in seven) are uninsured. First, Medicaid eligibility varies from state to state and, to keep costs down, some states have tightened up their criteria for eligibility so as to exclude many citizens. Second, many part-time workers in the service industries do not receive any benefits through their employment and cannot afford to take out expensive private insurance.

Spending on health care has run well ahead of inflation in recent decades

2o years p !

and cost containment has become a concern not only of governments but also of employers and insurers. A decade ago the federal government introduced the concept of Diagnostic Related Groups (DRGs) in an attempt to control Medicare hospital costs. Each in-patient was assigned to one of about 470 DRGs and the hospital received a fixed fee, regardless of the amount of treatment given. This had some effect on costs but led to increased use of out-patient and day care (styled ambulatory care) which did not come under the DRG system, and to some reduction in beds and hospitals as lengths of stay were reduced. HMOs and PPOs, often styled as 'managed care', have also been encouraged by governments as they are cheaper than traditional providers. Finally, in 1989 Congress legislated to introduce doctors' fee schedules following a detailed study of Relative Values which concluded that surgery fees in particular were normally far higher than was warranted. However, the new fees, which initially apply just to Medicare, only began to come into force in 1992, and will be phased in over several years.

Cost shifting has been another, and an unfortunate, feature of American cost containment. Insurers and Medicare and Medicaid programmes have increasingly expected patients to meet part of the costs of treatment through deductibles and co-payments. As a result some feel unable to afford needed care, and an estimated further 15 million are seriously underinsured, making some 50 million Americans (20 per cent of the population) either uninsured or underinsured.

Much of this activity to control costs reflects the private-sector basis of provision. Traditionally doctors and hospitals had determined their own prices, and fees were charged for each item of service provided. When Medicare and Medicaid were established (only in 1965) a deal was struck in the face of medical opposition – doctors retained the right to continue to charge their 'customary and prevailing' fees, a political decision which led to an income (and a cost) explosion and which the 1989 fee schedules will possibly alter.

Item of service fees encourage activity – the more diagnostic tests, and the more treatments or operations, the higher the income. HMOs operate on the opposite basis of offering cover at a fixed price, a system known as 'capitation'. With more than 30 million enrolled, HMOs are increasingly favoured by large employers concerned about their share of rising health-care costs. At around 11 per cent of Gross National Product, health-care spending in 1989 was far higher in the USA than in any other country. The UK, in contrast, spent only 6 per cent and Germany 8 per cent.

Doctors are licensed by state boards, but this is normally a formality in the case of those trained within the USA. Essentially they are free to practise anywhere, with the result that in San Francisco there is one doctor to every 175 inhabitants, whereas in officially designated shortage areas (mostly very remote and rural) there is one to at least 3500 and often many more. In some, but only a very few, areas the total absence of doctors has forced the profession to agree to nurses and pharmacists being able to prescribe, though this is not widely known and is the antithesis of professional policy which aims to retain the medical monopoly over drug prescribing.

The Veterans and Indian services employ salaried doctors, as do many HMOs. But the vast majority of US doctors are self-employed. Many work both from their own offices and in hospitals, where they have admitting rights. Family (or generalist) practitioners are in short supply. US doctors have tended to specialize, particularly in various surgical areas. Patients can go straight to a specialist, and many families have 'their' obstetrician, gynaecologist, paediatrician, surgeon, and so on, each acting independently from the others.

The item of service basis for fees has given doctors high incomes as well as incentives to treat. Recent comparative data showed US doctors to be earning 5.1 times the national average wage, compared to 2.8 times in the median OECD country (OECD, 1990). German doctors were close behind at 4.8 times the average wage, but UK doctors were low paid in comparison, at only 2.4 times. There has been increasing concern about the consequences of the incentive to treat, which makes operations like hysterectomies, caesarian births and appendectomies several times more common in the USA than in Britain. This has led to the introduction and rapid expansion of peer or utilization review systems in an attempt to halt unnecessary treatment. Review, or medical audit, is the systematic analysis of patient care designed to ensure that good medical practice takes place and to improve the quality of care. However, US physicians have maintained their relative salary levels in recent decades despite these cost containment developments and despite a rapid increase in the numbers of doctors (from 1 per 1000 population in 1960 to 1 per 400 in 1990).

Though US doctors have become wealthy, not least with the introduction of millions of new elderly and poor patients after the 1965 creation of Medicare and Medicaid, they have been less successful in retaining their individual clinical freedom. Peer and utilization review systems force doctors to justify, through detailed case notes, their treatment plans. Doctors, in effect, may have someone looking over their shoulder most of the time. This is not a mere formality as there are specialist private-sector utilization review corporations employed on the basis that the expenditure on them will be more than met by the reduced doctor and hospital bills which they obtain. Their livelihood depends on their reducing treatments. Medicare and Medicaid offices are now also becoming much more vigilant. Finally, the number of malpractice suits heard by the courts shows no sign of abating, and awards remain very high. Doctors have to pay large premiums to insure against such suits – up to one hundred times larger than in neighbouring Canada or in the UK where litigation is comparatively rare.

THE UNITED KINGDOM: A NATIONAL HEALTH SERVICE SYSTEM

In sharp contrast to the USA, the UK has one single dominant system of health care: its National Health Service, funded and run by government. Since 1948 the NHS has offered care to all which is free when received and paid for largely out of general taxation. Because the wealth of the patient plays no part in entitlement, access is formally dependent only on the need for treatment. That is the formality: in practice there is rationing through mechanisms like queuing – a non-urgent operation may necessitate a wait of several weeks or months, for example.

It is possible to pay for health care in the UK, and some do. But the private sector is small, accounting for only a little over 10 per cent of health spending. It is largely restricted to the extremely wealthy and to some managers where firms provide the premiums for an insurance policy as a fringe benefit. Much of its activity is in the provision of non-urgent surgery, where the NHS has a waiting list.

In the UK, then, government is to all intents and purposes both the payer and the provider of health care. The Department of Health has to annually negotiate funds with The Treasury, and the future level of spending is announced as part of government's general public expenditure programme. Health thus competes for funding with education, defence, social security and the many other areas of government activity, while the Chancellor of the Exchequer will seek to control any tax increases which might have to follow higher allocations to these public services. There are two consequences of this process. First, spending on the NHS has to be kept within a fixed budget and so is quite tightly controlled by the central government. Second, the competition between spending ministries for scarce resources is intense and not all requests for additional funds are met by the Chancellor – hence there is a common complaint from the NHS, voiced through its management and its staff, that more money should be spent on it. International comparisons are often cited: the less than 6 per cent of total national production spent annually on health care does place the UK, for better or worse, well down the league table of spending levels.

Though not a high spender in international terms, the UK Government is no different from other countries in its concern about rising costs. In the 1980s reforms were introduced designed to make the NHS more business-like, notably through the creation of General Managers, a concept borrowed from industry. In 1989 further and more far-reaching proposals were announced. These aim to introduce competition between NHS institutions, and involve creating an 'internal market' where NHS hospitals seek contracts to provide services to NHS purchasing boards. Providers and payers will be separated under this scheme, even though they both are part of the NHS.

This separation of providers and payers is possible because the NHS is not, and has never been, a single organization. Indeed, a distinguishing feature of the Service is just the opposite: administrative fragmentation. The central Department of Health acts as a sort of ringmaster. Fourteen Regional Health Authorities (RHAs) in England report directly to it (in Wales, Scotland and Northern Ireland there are different structures which add to the fragmentation). These RHAs are like the Department in that they also do not directly provide services to patients. Under the RHAs come the local boards primarily responsible for health care: some 190 District Health Authorities (DHAs) which oversee hospitals and community nurses, and 90 Family Health Services Authorities (FHSAs) which oversee the work of general medical practitioners, dentists, opticians and pharmacy shops. To this three tier–four organization structure have been added two new bodies under the 1989 reforms. First, individual hospitals and community units have been encouraged by the Government to break away from 'their' DHA and set up their own management, known as an NHS Trust. The DHA Purchasing Board may contract to receive services either from local Trusts, or from its own hospitals if these are still directly managed, or from hospitals or Trusts of other DHAs. Second, some large groups of General Practitioners have been encouraged to opt to become 'fund-holders'. They receive a budget which enables them (rather than the DHA Purchasing Board) to buy certain hospital services for their patients from wherever they think appropriate.

The distinction between DHAs and FHSAs reflects a division of labour agreed a century ago by the medical profession. FHSAs contract for the provision of primary care with individual general practitioners (GPs), who are self-employed. All patients register with a GP not just to receive primary care but because the GP alone can give the patient access to a hospital-based specialist (the only other route into hospital care is through the casualty or emergency department). There is no direct patient access to an NHS specialist, and this is a fundamental feature of the NHS which results in the vast bulk of doctor–patient activity taking place in the offices of GPs, who number about half the medical profession.

Though GPs are self-employed they have restrictions on both their mobility and their incomes. Geographical rationing is strong, and controlled by a national committee. This ensures that the ratio of patients to GPs is reasonably similar all over the country, and can prevent a GP from setting up in many areas unless there is a death or retirement.

Income is dominated by capitation – the GP contracts with the NHS to provide all necessary care for a fixed sum per patient which is determined by government after consultations and negotiations with the profession.

Hospital doctors, unlike GPs, are salaried. However, under an agreement made to overcome medical opposition to state control when the NHS was established in 1948, hospital doctors do not have to work full-time for the NHS. Salaries may thus be supplemented by private practice earnings, and senior specialists (known as 'consultants') frequently treat patients in private offices, private hospitals, or even in private beds within their NHS hospital for part of the week. Unlike GPs, they are not geographically constricted by a national medical manpower committee. However, mobility is severely affected by the national allocation of the numbers of consultants and of fixed financial budgets to RHAs, which in turn make fixed financial allocations to DHAs. Top–down decisions on resources thus in effect prevent any hospital from undertaking a major expansion of services, unless this has been planned through agreements with the higher authorities and contracts with DHA Purchasing Boards and GP Fundholders.

Despite the apparently complex and fragmented organizational structure of the NHS, doctors retain a great deal of clinical freedom. Systems known elsewhere as peer review or utilization review are little developed in the UK, and are only now beginning to be introduced under the title of 'medical audit'. Second opinions are rarely sought by hospital consultants, though the system of GP referral of patients to a hospital specialist could be said in itself to be a form of second opinion. This is not to say that doctors have total freedom of action, however, for the fixed NHS budget acts as a limitation. The UK doctor's individual clinical freedom is restricted not primarily by the need for peer accountability but rather by the resources available.

The NHS can thus allow its hospital doctors to continue to have the appearance of clinical freedom in the certain knowledge that medical colleagues will soon bring into line any consultant who introduces new forms of treatment which are expensive and which eat into the health-care budget. It can allow its GPs their clinical freedom because the capitation system gives them little or no incentive to treat patients solely to earn money (this argument applies also to salaried hospital doctors), and the only major additional drain on NHS funds has been through the open-ended freedom of GPs over the prescribing of medicines. Under the 1989 reform proposals an attempt has been made to curtail spending on drugs by giving GPs indicative drug budgets in order to make them fully aware of the costs to the NHS which they incur whenever they write out a prescription for a patient.

GERMANY: A COMPULSORY INSURANCE SYSTEM

The German health-care system has three significant features: the importance of compulsory insurance in funding health care; the variety of institutions concerned with care; and the roles played by government in the health-care system.

In Germany most medical care is free at the point of treatment; citizens rarely pay anything above a small sum when they consult a doctor, enter hospital or collect a prescribed drug from a pharmacist. Almost everybody in work is obliged to pay a health insurance premium. This in turn covers the cost of care for the contributor and for dependants. The significance of compulsory insurance is twofold. First, it is not confined to Germany; she pioneered this method of organizing health-care finance, and has been followed by many other nations. The country is thus the most important representative of this particular method of financing health care. Second, the way health insurance is run in Germany provides a set of institutions central to the nation's health-care system.

Compulsory insurance is not administered by the state. It is run by the health insurance funds. These funds are both compulsory and comprehensive, but there exist a strikingly large number to choose from – presently more than 1100. Each fund sets its own contribution rate, and each is obliged by law to raise the money needed to pay for the medical care given to its members. As a result, rates can differ between funds, since the costs of care will vary with the health-care demands of members.

Although it is usual to describe the German as an *insurance system*, the label is partly a misnomer, for two reasons. First, the 'premium' is in reality a payroll tax which the state obliges workers and employers to contribute. Second, although different funds set different contribution rates, the rate levied is the same for each member of a fund. This means that the amount an individual pays has nothing to do either with health risks faced by that individual, or with the calls he or she has made on the fund in the past. The key features of a true insurance system – that contribution rates are determined by risk and by the demand for cover – are thus absent. German and US arrangements can look superficially alike because they are conventionally described as two kinds of insurance system; but in reality, health-care funding in Germany is closer to the UK than to the US model, because it levies what is in effect a tax, and because most health care is given free at the point of treatment.

Not only are there many funds; there is great variety in the way they are organized. The most important group are district funds. As the name implies these are based on territory. District funds are separate, self-governing institutions, but they are also grouped into associations at both the national level and at the level of the individual states (*Länder*) who make up the

Federal Republic. (As we will see in Chapter 5, associations at the state – Länder – level are important in pay negotiations with doctors.) Other funds, by contrast, are based on occupation not territory. Here too there is variety. Some occupations, like civil servants, are served by a single nationwide fund. There also exists, however, a large number of so called factory funds based, as the name implies, on the individual workplace. To compound the variety there are some special funds for particular occupations, often surviving as historical legacies from the nineteenth century origins of the funding system.

Many workers can choose between funds, and there exists a limited amount of competition for members. The district funds, because they cover the whole country, are open to all workers. Whether an individual sub-scribes to a district fund, or to a fund designed for his or her occupation, is thus a matter of comparing the contribution rates levied by the competitors, and the detailed benefits that they offer.

The large number of funds, the different principles on which they are organized, and the many different associations into which they are grouped, all contribute to a complicated and decentralized health-care system. Decentralization and complexity are made more marked still by the part played by government in health care.

Although only about one-eighth of current health-care spending in Germany is accounted for by public institutions, government is the regulator of the whole health-care system. It is the source of 'compulsion' in the compulsory scheme of health insurance, because the power of the health insurance funds to impose levies on the workforce rests on legislation. The rules under which the parties to health care – insurance funds, doctors, patients – operate is contained in a succession of laws, starting with the sickness insurance legislation of 1883 which originally established the system. Government also supplies many of the basic resources for delivering health care: it has been the chief funder of hospital building; and it helps train doctors, who are mostly educated in state-funded universities.

Hence government unites the many institutions in Germany into a health-care system because it is the source of rules governing relations between the various parties, like doctors, patients and insurers. But as well as uniting, it also contributes to complexity and fragmentation. This is principally due to the federal organization of government in Germany. In the Federal Republic authority is distributed between Federal government in Bonn and the governments of the 16 individual states.

Government in the capital has little direct responsibility for delivering health care or for raising money to pay for care. Its importance lies in two spheres: federal laws provide the framework within which organizations like the insurance funds operate; and since any fundamental change in the health-care system requires a change in the legislative framework at the federal level, it is in Bonn that many of the most important debates about health-care policy take place. But some of the most important levers of policy are in the hands of the state (Länder) governments. The Länder control large parts of the hospital sector. They also control higher education in Germany – and this means that they have a large say over access to medical education and, thus, to the labour market for doctors. The federal system means that there is not one government concerned with health care, but 17 – the government in the capital and the governments in the individual states.

But even this does not exhaust the range of government bodies concerned with the regulation of the health-care system. The courts are also important. The powers of government in Germany are defined by the constitution – the so-called 'Basic Law'. It is the job of the courts, especially of the federal constitutional court, to interpret this constitution – to adjudicate when there are disputes about the allocation of power between the federal government and the states, and to adjudicate when there are disputes about what government in general is empowered to do. The constitutional court has made a number of important interventions in health-care policy by defining what government bodies, both in Bonn and in the Länder, can and cannot do in making policy. As we will see in Chapter 5, its decisions have been especially important in regulating access to the labour market for doctors.

The issues which have dominated debate about health-care policy in Germany are, not surprisingly, connected to the basic principles of the compulsory insurance system and to the way it is administered. Three are especially important. The first concerns the cost of care. Germany's spending on health care is not high by international standards, when the great wealth of the country is borne in mind. None the less, like most other nations she has seen spending grow fast in recent decades. This rise is reflected in the changing size of the 'premium' levied by the insurance funds: at the start of the 1970s the average for all employees was just over 8 per cent of income; by the end of the 1980s it was over 12 per cent. Since the middle of the 1970s there has been a continuous search for measures of 'cost containment'. Many of these, as we will see in Chapter 5, have affected doctors.

A second important issue is also related to the cost of care. It concerns, not the total bill, but the way the burdens and benefits of care are distributed in the population. The issue of burdens is connected to the way the insurance system is organized. Each fund sets its own contribution at the level needed to cover the cost of buying care for its members. These rates vary strikingly: at the extremes, the most heavily burdened funds levy a rate of 16 per cent, the most lightly burdened barely half this. They vary for two main reasons. Some funds have healthier members than others, and therefore have to find less to pay for care. And some funds have better paid members than others, and can therefore set low premiums because the 'tax base' is high. The higher contribution rates are concentrated in some of the 'district' funds covering the poorer parts of Germany. A percentage levy on the wages of poor people obviously yields less than does the same levy on the wages of rich people. The issue, in short, is that the contribution system is inegalitarian. The distribution of some health-care facilities is also inegalitarian. The geographical distribution of doctors, for instance, favours rich over poor communities (see Chapter 5): doctors prefer working in districts where the prosperous live than in, for instance, impoverished parts of cities.

Alongside these concerns about costs and benefits stands an issue about the capacity of the health-care system to deal with the question of reform. This is part of a wider debate about the organization of decision making in the Federal Republic. Some observers of German politics argue that decisive reform is especially difficult precisely because power is widely distributed between different institutions, allowing numerous organizations the chance to veto reform proposals (Katzenstein, 1987). Health care in Germany illustrates this wide distribution of powers and functions: the government in Bonn, the 16 Länder (states), the courts, the insurance funds and their organizations, the doctors' organizations: all have a say.

The issues of cost containment, distribution and the capacity to reform have been made more serious by the unification in 1990 of the two formerly separate German countries. This unification amounted to the abolition of the German Democratic Republic in the east, and the extension into the eastern territory of the institutions and practices of West Germany. Although change is only just beginning, some developments important for health-care policy can already be seen.

At the start of 1991 the health insurance system of the previous German Democratic Republic, which was run by a state institution, was replaced by a system of funds based on the model of the Federal Republic. The aim is to extend the structures, the entitlements and the rules of payment prevailing in the former 'West' Germany to the new territories. But this transition will take time, both because institutions cannot be built immediately, and because economic conditions are so different in the east. In particular, unemployment is high and wages are low. The funds in the east are running at a deficit, and have at the moment to be supported by public subsidy. How to even the enormous disparities in health-care financing between the former East and West Germanies will be a key issue in the years to come.

CONCLUSION

Doctors have many different roles, and operate in very different environments. From the point of view of regulation the doctor is far more than a physician: he or she is also both an economic actor with skills to sell and, commonly, a member of a pressure group with interests to defend. And, as the preceding sketches show, these different roles are performed in varying national settings. The three health-care systems that provide our examples exhibit many differences, and share many similarities.

The most important differences are threefold. The first and most obvious concerns the basic principle on which access to health care for individual citizens is regulated. The big division here is between the USA and the two other systems. In the UK and Germany, though the formal principles differ, the everyday experience for patients is basically similar: free, or virtually free, care at the point of treatment is an assured right. In the USA, by contrast, access to care is governed by different rules for different sections of the population. Three broad categories exist: those who have full, or fairly full, insurance bought in the marketplace; those who have some entitlements under a government scheme like Medicare; and those who have no cover at all.

A second key difference lies in the way the money to pay for health care is raised. Here the division is along different lines: Germany and the USA stand in contrast to the UK. In the UK the most striking feature is the overwhelming reliance on public money raised out of general taxation. In both the USA and Germany the most striking feature is the way the cost is spread among different parties. In the USA, about 40 per cent comes from government; the rest is spread between employers, insurance companies and private citizens. In Germany, just under half of the total spending on health is provided by the health insurance funds; the rest is spread between groups like government bodies, employers and private citizens.

A third key difference again separates the UK from our other two examples. Although the structure of the UK National Health Service is complicated, in England at any rate it is marked by a high degree of central control. In the USA and Germany, by contrast, what is remarkable is how far government authority is scattered in many different institutions, some at national, some at sub-national levels.

We will see that all these differences affect the regulation of the medical profession in our three countries. But the features uniting the three are also remarkable. In all three medicine is 'big business', measured either by the numbers involved in health care or by the sums of money spent. In all three, the issue of cost, and in particular of rising costs, is central to debates about health-care policy. And in all three doctors are a key part of the health-care system – in delivering care, in allocating resources, and in consuming resources themselves. In other words, the regulation of doctors is a key to the way all three health-care systems function – and it is to regulation that we now turn.

FURTHER READING

An outstanding account of the historical development of the US medical profession is Starr (1982). Alford (1975) offers a framework by seeing physicians as the key group in the politics of health in the USA, placing them in context as one of three interests (the corporate rationalizers and consumers are the other two. Fox (1987) compares and contrasts UK and US twentieth century public debates and policies on health care. Allsop (1984) looks briefly into the history of the UK medical profession in chapter 2, and German developments are best outlined for readers of English by Murswieck (1985), Oppl and von Kordoff (1990) and Iglehart (1991a, b).

The US health-care system is outlined in some detail in Raffel and Raffel (1989) while Gray (1983) considers the rise of state action and response of physicians. The best texts on the UK are Ham (1992), Klein (1989) and Harrison *et al.* (1990). On the German system, see Alber (1991) for the most up-to-date sketch.

The UK reforms of 1989–91 are put into a comparative context by Ham *et al.* (1990) whose text includes separate chapters on seven countries, including the USA and Germany. In the 1980s pioneering attempts at comparative analysis based on statistical data were made by the OECD (1990), whose publications include important non-statistical cross-national reviews of different health-care systems in action. Schieber *et al.* (1991) use the OECD database to discuss, *inter alia*, the supply, workload and costs of physicians in almost all the 26 developed countries of the world.

For readers of German, the best introduction to the German system is Alber (1989), which 'sets' the health-care system in the context of the wider welfare state.

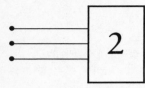

THE STATE, PROFESSIONS AND REGULATION

INTRODUCTION

This chapter is designed to introduce the reader to the study of regulation. The regulation of doctors obviously has its own special features. But to treat the regulation of the medical profession as simply something special to medicine is to miss a key feature: doctors are regulated in societies where numerous other occupations and markets are also regulated. And it transpires that the regulation of doctors has much in common with the task of regulation in other parts of the modern economy. The chapter therefore starts with an examination of the nature of regulation in general. It then focuses on the special features of *professional regulation*, examining in particular the debate about the distinguishing features of a profession. Finally, it concentrates on the case of doctors as a regulated profession, identifying the recent debates about regulation and the power of doctors. By the end of the chapter the reader should be able to turn to the historical evidence about the development of regulation in the medical profession equipped with a basic knowledge about the general character of regulation as an activity, and with a knowledge of the main debates about the nature of professional regulation in medicine.

THE NATURE OF REGULATION

What should medical students be taught in order to qualify as doctors? Who should run medical education? How should doctors be paid? What controls are needed over the way they do their job?

Every reader will recognize that these questions are central to the lives of doctors – and to the lives of their patients. They encapsulate some of the key issues which have to be settled in the *regulation* of the medical profession. But they are not peculiar to medicine. The needs of medicine of course demand special arrangements, but there is nothing unique about the general problems involved in regulating the medical profession, nor about the way those problems are solved. Doctors provide a service, and regulating the supply of that service poses issues similar to the regulation of any other good or service supplied in the community.

The issues can be summarized as those concerning *standards, accountability* and *efficiency*. Any system of regulation has to say something about the standards of technical competence and ethical probity which will be demanded of practitioners; any system of regulation has to decide if practitioners will be obliged to give an account of their actions, and if so to whom; and any system of regulation likewise has to decide how far, if at all, it will be concerned with the efficiency and effectiveness with which practitioners deliver a service. We will discover that while these issues are particularly important in the regulation of doctors, they crop up, not only in medicine, but in regulation as a whole.

Regulation is the activity by which the rules governing the exchange of goods and services are made and implemented. We can see immediately that it is the foundation of social life. Every kind of market has to be regulated. Making and selling cars; supplying banking services; delivering personal services as varied as hairdressing or burial of the dead: all these take place within a framework of rules. The study of regulation examines how these rules come about, how they are implemented and how the institutions responsible for making and implementing rules come into existence and operate.

The activity of regulation can in turn be broken down into four separate tasks: the control of market entry and exit, of competitive practices, of market organization and of remuneration. These tasks have to be carried out regardless of whether the activity in question is the provision of doctoring or the sale of automobiles.

The *regulation of market entry* is the first task that has to be performed, because the first questions that have to be answered in regulation are: who can engage in the activity, and what conditions must they meet in order to have the right to do the job? Rules of market entry vary from the highly permissive to the exceptionally restrictive: almost anybody can set up as a window cleaner, whereas to become a banker or a lawyer involves meeting stringent standards set and enforced by specialized regulatory bodies. One of the central tasks in the study of regulation is to understand why there exists this spectrum from permissiveness to restrictiveness, and to discover how far it can be explained by the needs of the activity being regulated.

The second task, the *regulation of competitive practices*, arises because most societies allow competition in the provision of goods and services, but all place limits on the extent of that competition. Some limits are set by laws concerned with the overall organization of economic life: thus laws against fraud and theft, and laws enforcing freely made contracts, are all designed to restrict the exploitation of the honest by the dishonest. Within this general framework of regulation, however, almost all goods and services are subject to more particular rules: drugs may not be marketed by pharmaceutical companies until they have satisfied safety tests; cigarettes can only be marketed with a health warning, while their advertisement is restricted in some countries and banned in others; and in some countries particular occupational groups – like lawyers – are prohibited from competing for business by advertising their services.

The third task is related to the control of competitive practices, but it deserves separate examination. The *regulation of market structures* is necessary because markets have to be organized: decisions need to be made about what kinds of institutions will be allowed to provide goods and services. For instance, most nations have rules governing mergers and takeovers of private firms; these in effect control the conditions under which the structure of ownership in markets can be changed. In some cases regulation actually prohibits some organizations and prescribes others: for example, until recently UK solicitors could not organize their business in companies enjoying limited liability. In some parts of the insurance business, for instance, it is only possible to engage in business through partnerships rather than through companies enjoying limited liability. Some regulations prescribe upper and lower limits to the size of firms in a market: most banking regulation demands that banks have minimum reserves of capital. In many countries anti-monopoly rules forbid single firms from controlling more than a prescribed percentage of production or sales in a particular market. Market structure regulation also tries to influence the distribution of suppliers. In some instances geographical distribution is regulated: the urban planning system in the UK limits the numbers of particular kinds of shops that can be established in a district; while in the USA most banks are prohibited from operating networks of branches that cross state boundaries.

The fourth and final task that has to be performed is *the regulation of payment*. In any transaction some rules always exist about payment for the good or service being exchanged, even if these rules are only the general framework provided by laws for enforcing contracts and curbing fraud. In many cases there exist more detailed rules governing both scales of charges and actual methods of charging. In professions like law it is common to find fixed scales of charges. In some markets, payment is by collective bargaining between providers and payers; the classic cases lie in labour markets where unions bargain over pay with representatives of employers. At the other extreme – consider the local window cleaner or the haggling that goes on in a used-car showroom – it is the result of an individual deal between the customer and the provider. There are thus great variations in how far payment is regulated: but some decision about the extent and form of regulation has to be made, even if the decision amounts to leaving the customer and supplier free to haggle.

The four tasks outlined here have to be performed in some way in all markets. Their relevance to the medical profession should be clear. In organizing its medical profession each country has to make decisions about the following: how applicants who enter medicine are screened and trained; how far, once in, they will be allowed to compete for business, and what ethical standards will govern their relations with clients; in what institutional settings – hospitals, their own consulting rooms – doctors can practise their profession; and how doctors will be paid? The 'special' problems of regulating doctors are, in other words, only particular instances of the more general problems of regulation.

Of course doctors are not in the marketplace in exactly the same way as window cleaners, bankers or used-car salesmen. On the contrary, one of the distinctive features of medicine as an occupation lies in how far commercial competition is restricted. As we will see in the next section, these controls are often thought to be one of the marks that single out medicine as a *profession*. The controls are the result of particular solutions to the four regulatory tasks identified above. The solutions vary between countries, and have varied over time. There is no single 'model' of regulation – and the pattern in any one country is certainly not the only model. The following illustrations give some indication of the variety.

Entry regulation into the medical profession takes many forms. Acquiring a licence to practise medicine commonly demands acceptance into, and completion of, extended courses in medical education and long periods of practical training but the exact requirements vary from country to country. Most nations – and all those considered in this text – also have their own distinctive rules controlling entry to particular specialisms. In brief, every nation gives an elaborate but different answer to the question: who can become a doctor?

Regulation of competitive practices has been virtually one of the defining features of medicine as a modern profession. As we will see in Chapter 3 there is a long history of efforts to distinguish the doctor from providers of other commercial services. This often took the form of putting limits on competition for patients, and providing 'consumer protection' in the form of ethical codes governing the relations between doctor and patient. All modern health-care systems now have rules restricting, and in some cases prohibiting, advertisements for business by doctors; all regulate the freedom of patients to choose or change doctors; and all have rules governing the personal relations between doctor and patient.

These rules often overlap with *the regulation of market structures.* The practice of medicine has to be organized in some institutions, whether the institution is the 'solo' doctor operating a one-person business or a health service employing all doctors as public servants. The way it should be organized has provided, and continues to provide, some of the most difficult of regulatory issues. For most of this century the preferred solution was to treat the doctor as a species of independent businessman, operating as a 'solo practitioner'. But 'solo practitioners' have always operated alongside other parts of the health-care system, like hospitals. One of the thorniest issues has been the proper division of labour between doctors working inside, and those working outside, hospitals – an issue which, as we shall see, has been settled differently in the three countries examined in this book. More recently, the very idea of the 'solo practitioner' – the doctor operating as a kind of small business – has been challenged by the spread of other ways of organizing the provision of medical services: for instance, by the practice of employing doctors for a salary in profit or non-profit making institutions. The issue of doctors' freedom to operate as independent entrepreneurs does not, however, exhaust the range of problems involved in the regulation of market structures. Among the remainder, one that will recur in these pages is regulation of the geography of markets. It is common for systems to operate some restrictions over where doctors may follow their profession. There is also a continuing debate about how far existing regulations adequately distribute doctors to those areas where they are most needed.

Finally, *payment regulation* is perhaps the most important and controversial task in the regulation of the medical profession. All regulatory systems have to make some decision about what financial relationship, if any, is to exist between the patient and the doctor. The possibilities can be placed on a spectrum. At one end the doctor sets the fee for treatment in the manner of any other private entrepreneur offering a service, and the regulation of payment amounts to no more than the imposition of general rules governing the carrying out of contractual obligations in a market. In the past this was the usual way to regulate payment in many health-care systems; now it is rare. At the other end of the spectrum, no money changes hands at the moment of treatment, and payment is funded by some third party – the government from the public purse, or a health insurance company or fund. In practice, as we will see, none of the health-care systems studied in this book is at either extreme end of the spectrum. Each uses some mixture of direct payment by the patient and some sort of payment by an institution – though the bulk of payments come from institutions rather than directly from patients in the surgery.

The question of who pays the doctor is, however, not the only important issue in the regulation of remuneration. Just as significant is the way payment is calculated. Again it is helpful to visualize the possibilities along a spectrum. At one end is pure 'payment per service': every possible service that the doctor can perform is costed according to some kind of scale of fees, and the amount paid is simply a result of the sum of services performed for every patient. At the other end of the spectrum is a pure salary system: the doctor is paid a fixed income irrespective of the number of patients seen or the treatments they receive. As we will yet again see, none of the countries examined in the succeeding pages is at either extreme on the spectrum, but they are all at different points along that spectrum.

The comparative study of the regulation of the medical profession examines how the four regulatory tasks sketched here are performed in different countries, and tries to explain differences and similarities. In part this is a matter of looking at the substance of the rules governing market entry, competitive practices, market structure and pay. But alongside the important matter of the *substance* of rules are two further equally important sets of questions: about *procedures and processes* – in other words about how rules are made and put into effect; and about *outcomes* – who gets what out of the regulatory system.

The most important factor we consider hinges on the role of the state in the regulation of doctors. When we look at the way regulation is actually carried out in any particular instance we find that it usually involves many different principles of organization. But the many different combinations are based on three broad ways of organizing regulation. The three allocate different roles to the state. They are: independent self-regulation; state sanctioned self-regulation; and state administered regulation.

Under *independent self-regulation* those concerned with an activity solve the main regulatory tasks independently of the state. This does not necessarily mean that free-market forces are allowed to decide how a good or service is provided. On the contrary, those engaged in a trade or profession may well erect elaborate controls over market entry and competitive practices. In modern society this sort of pure self-regulation is actually quite rare in any important sector of the economy, simply because the modern state is seldom content to leave regulation totally in private hands. Nowadays the best examples of 'pure' models of independent self-regulation are to be found in the fields of leisure, culture and religion. It is common for sporting associations, bodies for the promotion of the arts, and churches, to organize their affairs as purely private associations. Even here, however, independence is on the decline: in recent years in the UK, for instance, the internal conduct of the sport of soccer has increasingly been subject to government control.

This example gives us a hint of how independent self-regulation can turn into *state-sanctioned self-regulation*. The essence of the difference is immediately apparent: in the latter the rules, and the institutions concerned with their formulation and implementation, exist with the consent and support of the state and, in the last analysis, are operated with the support of state sanctions. In recent decades state sanctioning has increasingly displaced pure independent self-regulation. In many cases existing regulatory institutions have been brought under state supervision, while retaining the function of carrying out the detailed tasks of regulation. 'Self-regulation in a statutory framework' is now the standard method of organization in, for example, financial markets in the UK, where a series of 'self-regulatory organizations' control insurance, stock exchanges and allied markets under powers delegated from central government. Likewise many occupations regulate their own arrangements under powers delegated from the state. On the continent of Europe this pattern of self-regulation is especially common. Many regulatory institutions on the continent, especially in the business community, are public law bodies, operated by their own members but endowed with the powers of public agencies.

State-sanctioned self-regulation is widespread for a variety of reasons. In many cases it developed out of older systems of independent self-regulation, when failures in the old arrangements led to reform and state supervision. This is how, for instance, traditional systems of independent self-regulation in the financial markets of the UK and of the USA developed into state-sanctioned self-regulation: in both countries fraud and financial collapse led to demands that government supervise and license the institutions doing the job of regulation. Using the state in this way solves a number of problems simultaneously. Genuinely independent self-regulation often faces serious problems of control, because it is difficult for voluntary associations to wield sanctions against those who break rules. Putting state power behind the system can supply the necessary authority. At the same time, by delegating to private bodies the detailed tasks of regulation states are saved the considerable financial and administrative burden of doing the jobs themselves.

This kind of state licensing poses considerable problems of accountability. By licensing a private body to carry out regulatory functions in its name, the state gives power to that body. The conditions under which that power is granted – the extent to which delegated powers are subject to scrutiny and review, the amount of authority delegated, the powers of punishment devolved – are critical to the functioning of state-sanctioned self-regulation.

State-sanctioned self-regulation in practice 'shades into' the third system identified above, *direct state regulation*. The identifying features of the latter are as follows. Authority to regulate rests on legislation. Regulation may be carried out by a specialized public institution, or by a group of civil servants in a central department of government. The principles of the system are that those who make the rules, and those who implement them, are public servants: they are employees of the state, are subject to rules of public accountability and their actions can be reviewed and challenged in the courts. In principle, direct state regulation ensures public accountability; how far it does so in practice is a matter for investigation of particular cases.

Independent self-regulation, state-sanctioned self-regulation and direct state regulation are three different ways by which the regulatory tasks sketched earlier in this chapter can be carried out. In the UK case, for instance, we will discover that there is a bias towards state-sanctioned self-regulation, though this does not rule out the use of the other forms. There is no reason to assume, however, that other countries share this bias – nor, indeed, that they use one form of regulation to the exclusion of others. The purpose of examining regulation comparatively is to discover the differences between nations, and if possible to explain those differences. In Figure 2.1 we provide a simple 'matrix' of the possibilities which have emerged from the discussion so far.

The organization of regulation

The regulatory tasks				
	Market entry	Competitive practices	Market structures	Remuneration
Independent self-regulation				
State-sanctioned self-regulation				
Direct state regulation				

Figure 2.1 The regulatory matrix.

THE NATURE OF PROFESSIONAL REGULATION

Regulating doctors is in many ways like regulating other occupations. But doctors also have their own special features, and one reason they are special is that, almost everywhere, they are thought to belong to a distinctive category called *professions*. The regulation of the doctor is therefore an example of a particularly important kind of regulatory activity – professional regulation.

Although professions are acknowledged to be one of the most important occupational groups in modern economies, there is disagreement about how to recognize a profession. Three contrasting solutions exist: the normative approach, the 'trait' approach, and the occupational control approach.

The *normative* approach suggests that a profession is distinguished by a particularly well-developed ethical code. Occupations that, like medicine, aspire to professional status always develop such a code. Indeed medicine has, in the Hippocratic Oath, perhaps the oldest and most famous code. This suggests that the enforcement of particularly high ethical standards is what marks it out as a profession. In the terms used in the previous section, a heavy emphasis is placed on *the regulation of competitive practices*, to protect clients or customers. One of the first influential studies of professions argued (Carr-Saunders and Wilson, 1933, quoted in Wilding, 1982, p. 13), for instance, that professions

> engender modes of life, habits of thought and standards of judgement which render them centres of resistance to crude forces which threaten steady and peaceful evolution.

There are two objections to identifying professions according to these normative standards. First, they take an occupation's own valuation of itself as definitive. It is conceivable, after all, that ethical codes exist to do more than protect clients: for instance, to limit competition and to raise the incomes of the members of the profession. A second objection is that the normative solution is not good at discriminating between occupations. A huge range of trades, from brain surgery to second-hand car selling, employ some sort of code; but a category that lumps together such a wide range is not illuminating. If almost any conceivable trade can be a profession by announcing that it has an ethical code, then the category loses its value as a way of distinguishing a particular kind of regulation.

Since one of the drawbacks of the normative approach is that it selects only one feature as a defining mark of professional status, an obvious alternative is to look for a bundle of features. This is the thought that lies behind what both Johnson (1972) and Wilding (1982) call the 'trait approach' – the approach that searches for a range of characteristics which, put together, make an occupation a profession (for example, traits like nature of work, methods of entry). Wilding has also identified the key difficulty with the trait approach: in practice, attempts by students of professionalism to identify the key traits have shown that there is no consensus over what these are. The trait approach could only work in two circumstances. We could develop an abstract 'ideal' of a profession composed of a collection of traits – in which case we have simply moved back to the normative approach to identification. Alternatively, we could look at the range of occupations that claim professional status and try to identify what they have in common. But it is precisely this latter approach which has failed to produce a consensus. Nor is the lack of consensus surprising. Even within a single field like medicine the range of jobs claiming professional title is very wide. Leaving aside the obvious case of the various kinds of doctors, we also have chiropodists, physiotherapists, radiographers and ophthalmic opticians (Larkin, 1983). Beyond medicine, identifying a common set of traits uniting insurance brokers, accountants, sanitary engineers and clergymen is highly problematical.

So many different groups claim professional status that we will probably find it impossible to distil the common features that unite them. But this very diversity can be turned to good account, because it suggests a third solution to the problem of identification. The fact that so many occupations claim to be professions shows that professionalism is a highly desired status. It is highly desired in part because, whatever the reality, professionalism is associated in the minds of many with rigorous standards of ethics and competence. Labelling an occupation a 'profession' thus immediately raises its standing in the eyes both of practitioners and of the community. But according to some theorists it does more; it offers those who practise the occupation the chance more effectively to control the market for their services – and thus to increase power over clients and the rewards of the job. According to this view professionalism is not a set of traits which jobs have in common, nor a distinct ethic, but a mode of occupational control. It is a special way of regulating the market in the services offered by an occupation. 'A profession is not, then' to quote Johnson, 'an occupation but a means of controlling an occupation' (1972, p. 45). Occupations like medicine are in particular need of professional status, according to this view, because of the nature of the job. Medicine is an intrusive business, involving examination of the most intimate and sensitive matters. Ideas of professionalism – of special ethical codes, of unusual care of clients – help make intrusion acceptable.

Freidson has argued that medicine is a particularly striking example of professionalism as occupational control. And according to Freidson this occupational control is notably political, because it involves the profession in a contract with the most important of all political institutions – the state. He writes: (1970, p. xvii)

> It is useful to think of a profession as an occupation which has assumed a dominant position in the division of labour, so that it gains control over the determination of the substance of its own work.

One of the key ways modern professions accomplish this dominant position is by acquiring power and authority from the most important source of power and authority in modern societies – the state. In the case of medicine, the 'foundation of medicine's control over its work,' says Freidson, 'is thus clearly political in character, involving the aid of the state in establishing and maintaining the profession's pre-eminence' (1970, p. 23).

Thus professionalism, in the language of our preceding section, is a particular form of state-sanctioned, or state-licensed, regulation. Indeed, we will see in Chapter 3 that the history of regulation among doctors is precisely a history of the use of state power to license the profession's control over its activities.

Now that we have realized that professional regulation is based on a regulatory contract with the state, three important conclusions follow. First, politics lies at the heart of regulation. The regulation of medicine is not just a technical matter of setting standards. It is a political process, involving the exercise of power and authority in struggles between competing interests; and it is a process in which the struggle for control of state power is central. In Chapter 3 we will see that the historical development of medical regulation has indeed often been affected by the wider character of the state.

Secondly, we realize that the regulatory contract between the medical profession and the state can be negotiated very differently in different countries. If professionalism is a species of occupational control licensed by the state, the terms of the licence need not everywhere be the same, because states are not everywhere the same. We will see in later chapters that in some cases doctors have been given the 'licence' from the state with little public control or supervision; in others, state oversight and control is great.

A third conclusion is that not only will professional organization differ between countries; the substance of the rules can also vary. There is no single 'professional' way to perform the four regulatory tasks identified earlier: those of market entry, of competition, of market structures or of pay. Some professions, for instance, exercise tight control over the amount of competition between members; others allow extensive competition for business. In the UK, medicine has more restrictive rules than have architecture or accounting; and medicine in the UK has more restrictive controls than has the medical profession in the USA. A single profession can also alter its rules over time: the law in the UK used to allow very little competition; in recent years the rules have been relaxed. Changes over time are especially important for the medical profession. As we will see in the next section, some observers of medicine argue that doctors once enjoyed almost total command over their occupation, but that recent changes have forced them to share control with other interests.

Professionalism is a form of occupational control, a way of regulating the market in a job through controls over entry, over competitive practices, over market structures and over payment. This regulation is done with the agreement of the state, but the form of that agreement – the amount of state supervision, the exact content of rules – varies over time and in different countries. Before we describe in Chapter 3 how regulation has developed historically, we should look at the most important reasons for these variations.

THE DETERMINANTS OF REGULATION

Regulation is political: the institutions that develop, and the rules that those institutions enforce, are produced by the exercise of power. Relations of power are influenced by many factors, so regulation itself is determined by many factors. Out of a multitude of influences, however, three are especially important: the *place* where regulation is conducted; the *time* when it is conducted; and the nature of the *job* that is being regulated.

Place refers to the national setting of regulation. The regulation of doctors is conducted within the framework of different national political systems. National political systems obviously vary. Only three national political systems are represented in this book, but even these three show striking differences. The USA and Germany are both federal systems, while the UK has a unitary system of government. This means that, while in the UK political power and authority are concentrated on national government in London, in the USA and Germany much political power is located in the individual states who are members of the federation – states like California in the USA, or Länder (states) like Bavaria in Germany. And when we turn to look at doctors we will see that the institutions of regulation in the different countries do reflect this broader political difference: in Germany and the USA medical regulation has a much more federal character than in the UK.

The influence of federal as against unitary structures is only the most obvious example of how national setting can influence regulation. More subtle, but equally important, are different national ideas of the place of law in the regulatory sphere. Here again there is a striking contrast between, on the one hand, the UK, and on the other the USA and Germany. The first of these has no written constitution, and there has been a tendency to rely on informal understandings rather than on formally codified arrangements in regulation. In the USA and Germany, on the other hand, the existence of written constitutions has accompanied a stronger tendency to put down the details of regulation on the statute book. The most immediate result is that doctors in the UK have been able to practise without knowing much about the law; in the USA and Germany, knowing the law is more important. Likewise, nations differ in the way professions and the state have historically been related. Most work on professions, and therefore most theorizing about professions, is based on work done in the Anglo-Saxon world, especially in the USA and in the UK. These states, however, show a particular form of 'liberal' professionalism, under which professions have operated relatively independently of government. The state has allowed professions a high degree of independence. Germany has a different tradition, in which professions have been much more closely connected to the state. In the case of some professions – like teachers – this is reflected in the fact that they are employed as state bureaucrats.

The many differences in regulation between nations have been systematized by the American political scientist David Vogel into the argument that there exist distinctive *national styles of regulation*. Vogel (1986, pp. 267–8) writes:

> We can . . . distinguish roughly three broad national patterns of government regulation: The British, the continental, and the American.

The UK pattern, he argues,

> . . . differs sharply from the legal orientation of the continental nations, with their roots in the civil (Roman) law. The continental approach differs from that of Britain in its emphasis on precise rules and time-tables and centrally determined standards.

The US pattern is, he argues, also unique. It is distinctive

> . . . in the degree of oversight exercised by the judiciary and the national legislature, in the formality of its rule making and enforcement process, in its reliance on prosecution, in the amount of information made available to the public, and in the extent of the opportunities provided for participation by nonindustry constituencies.

The argument that there are distinct national styles of regulation suggests that in the regulation of the medical profession we should look, not for a single common medical pattern, but for variations dictated by the particular national setting in which regulation occurs. That is the most important reason why our discussion in this book is comparative.

But 'national style' cannot be the whole story: not every profession within a country has the same regulatory institutions, nor the same rules about entry or competing for business. Even if there do exist predominant national patterns, there are many variations on these patterns. One of the most important sources of these variations is the *timing* of regulation. Obviously not all systems of regulation develop simultaneously. We will see in Chapter 3 that regulation in medicine happened at different rates and in different periods in the three countries that concern us. Differences in timing open up a wide range of influences. 'Early' regulators, like the UK, can be copied by later regulators: some US regulation in medicine seems to have been directly copied from the UK. The content of regulation is often shaped by wider historical conditions which have no direct connection with medicine: we will see that in the case of Germany much of what now exists is the result of the country's turbulent political history after the Nazi seizure of power in the 1930s. More generally still, there is a powerful force for inertia in regulation. Institutions and rules developed in response to the needs of a particular time do not necessarily disappear when the historical conditions that produced them have vanished; they often continue into a very different historical period.

The regulation of doctors, like the regulation of other groups and interests, is undoubtedly influenced by the national setting in which regulation is conducted and by the historical period when the system of regulation was originally constructed. But regulation is also a product of more immediate forces that are special to the profession itself: in other words, the third influence identified above, *the nature of the job*, is important. In part this is a matter of the distinct demands of the professional task: because a doctor and an architect need different skills, this is going to affect the way the two professions are regulated. But it is also a matter of the way different professions have their own distinct internal systems of politics. Within any profession regulation is a continuing political process – the outcome of a constant series of decisions that result from competition between groups enjoying different amounts of power. The groups are different in architecture, in accountancy, in engineering – and in medicine. In the case of medicine the most important power groups include the different branches of the medical profession itself; the large business interests – like pharmaceutical companies – who produce and market medical goods and services; other occupations concerned with the provision of health care, like pharmacists and nurses; those who pay for health care, whether they are the patients themselves, insurance companies who provide cover for patients, or the government; and those who are the recipients of health care, the patients. All these groups have an interest in the regulation of doctors, but they do not all command the same amount of power; and the way regulation works is influenced by the particular balance of power between the different interests in the medical arena.

Attempts to identify the balance of power in medicine have produced a prolonged debate focused on the power of doctors. Three contrasting views are especially important.

The first is the *professional domination view*: this says that doctors themselves, organized as a profession, dominate regulation. A second view admits that doctors did once dominate, but argues that we are now seeing a process of *declining professional power*. Both these views assert that the distribution of power is roughly the same irrespective of the type of health-care system in which doctors operate – the first suggesting that they are everywhere dominant, the second that they are everywhere in decline. A third view argues, by contrast, that power is shaped by the organization of the *wider health-care system*.

The professional domination hypothesis has been argued with particular force by Freidson (1970). According to Freidson what we observe in the case of medicine is the successful control over a key part of the medical labour market by a particular occupational group, to the exclusion of other parties. This success is due to a combination of effective organization by doctors, the support from the state enjoyed by those organizations, and the ability of doctors to establish themselves as the custodians of medical knowledge. In short, regulation is a way by which the privileged position of doctors is established at the expense of other groups, whether patients or other providers of health care.

Against this view in recent years has been heard the argument that doctors' power in the regulatory process, though once great, is now in decline. Among advocates of the *declining professional power* view, however, there are significant differences of emphasis. One important account is derived from a US study that has proved widely influential. In an investigation of health-care policy making in New York, Alford (1975) distinguished three distinct sets of interests at work in the arena of medical politics. He labelled these the *dominant*, the *challenging* and the *suppressed*. The first corresponded to the most prestigious parts of the medical profession, which had once managed to monopolize control over health care. The second he identified with the 'corporate rationalizers' – health-care managers, and payers like insurance companies, who wished to reduce medical autonomy in the interests of efficiency and economy. The third, suppressed, interest included patients. Alford interpreted conflict over regulation as the result of the growing challenge posed by the corporate rationalizers. The growing cost of health care forced rationalizers to try to curb the freedom of doctors in order to get control over budgets and work practices.

A more emphatic account still argues, not just that doctors' power is being challenged, but that there is actually taking place a long-term decline in that power. Klein (1989) in his study of the UK, and Starr and Immergut (1987) in a comparative analysis of several countries, have both argued this proposition. According to Starr and Immergut, for example, there did exist a period in the fairly recent past – up to the beginning of the 1960s – when the medical profession was dominant. This coincided with a period of public confidence in the capacity of medicine to deliver good health. It also coincided with years of sustained economic growth that funded continuous increases in the resources given to medical care. In recent decades, however, there has occurred a long-term loss of public confidence in the medical profession's capacity to secure good health. In addition, the problem of cost containment has become acute in almost every nation. As the search for more economical ways of treatment has intensified, the payers – whether the state, private individuals, employers or insurers – have begun to question the right of doctors to make decisions without regard to considerations of cost and efficiency. A similar argument is advanced by Haug (1988), though she focuses more on the independence of the individual doctor at work than on relations between the organized profession and the state. According to Haug, patients are becoming more educated and more demanding, while knowledge of medicine and medical practices is becoming more widespread. Doctors are thus facing more assertive and challenging consumers of their services. Still other writers depict the change in the language of 'proletarianization'. McKinlay and Arches (1985) see a long-term loss of control by doctors over entry to medicine and a decline in the autonomy of the individual physician. These changes have been accompanied by 'deskilling', a process in which the job of the doctor is broken down into narrow specialisms which can increasingly be performed mechanically.

The advocates of the view that doctors are a dominant power, and of the alternative view that they are a declining power, share a common assumption that the power of the medical profession is more or less the same regardless of how the health-care system is organized. This is exactly what is questioned by the third view summarized here – which is that the organization of the health-care system itself significantly influences the distribution of power. However, two diametrically opposed versions of this view exist. Some argue that where the state rather than the market organizes the provision of health, the power of doctors is greatly diminished. When the state funds medical care, according to this view, it is bound to intervene increasingly in the affairs of the medical profession in order to influence what is happening to its money. It is precisely this fear of the power of the state under 'socialized medicine' which lies behind the opposition of much of the US medical profession to the introduction of a national health service or of national health insurance in that country. It was also the reasoning behind the unsuccessful opposition by many doctors to the introduction of the NHS into the UK at the end of the 1940s. The extreme example of this state domination can be found in the health-care systems that existed in eastern Europe before the great political changes of 1989–90. There, the state funded most health care and doctors were state employees. The rewards of medicine in these systems were also much less than in countries where the market was important: doctors in eastern Europe were generally paid less than many manual workers, whereas in the West they have generally been among the best paid professionals.

But an entirely contrasting view is put forward by some observers of the USA, which has a health-care system where the market remains especially important. According to this alternative argument the organization of the health-care system does indeed decide who has most influence in regulation; but the market system in the USA actually reduces, rather than enhances, the influence of the medical profession (Döhler, 1989). This is because in a market system those who have to pay for care – especially large employers who usually pick up the bill for the health insurance premiums of their employees – have a powerful incentive to intervene in regulation in order to try to contain costs. As we will see later in this book the recent history of payment regulation in the USA is indeed marked by growing control over the working practices of the individual doctor.

CONCLUSION

This chapter has shown that the regulation of doctors is part of a wider process of regulation that takes place in society. Medicine has its own special needs, and the medical arena has its own particular interests and power structures. These special features will exert a distinctive influence on the way any country regulates its own medical profession. But regulation here has important features in common with the regulation of other social arenas. There is a market for the services of doctors, and in all markets particular regulatory tasks have to be carried out: regulation of entry, of competition, of structure and of pay. Doctors do not perform these tasks in the same way as other occupations – but they have to perform them in some way, and we understand better how the medical profession functions if we have some understanding of the range of options that are in principle open to those regulating markets. Likewise doctors are a profession, and this feature deeply influences how physicians are regulated; but we understand the regulation of the medical profession better when we bear in mind that, for all its individualities, medicine is only one of a range of professional occupations, and the way medicine as a profession organizes itself is influenced by the wider pattern of professional regulation in society. For the doctor, regulation has two sides: on the one side, it is a source of restrictions and controls, but on the other, it is a source of opportunity – it provides security against competitors and the chance to organize the labour market. This tension between regulation as restriction, and regulation as opportunity, recurs throughout the following pages.

Now that we have placed doctors against the wider regulatory background, we must turn to a closer examination of how the regulation of the medical profession developed in the three countries that are examined in this study. That is the purpose of Chapter 3.

FURTHER READING

One of the first influential studies of the regulation of professions was Carr-Saunders and Wilson (1933). More recent general analyses are to be found in Freidson (1970), in Johnson (1972) and in Wilding (1982). Richman (1987), Chapter 5, reviews the debate about the professionalization of health care. Alford (1975) is now a modern classic on the 'challenge' to medical power. Vogel (1986) says nothing about medicine, but is the standard study of 'national styles' of regulation.

The regulation of medicine is examined comparatively by Starr and Immergut (1987). On the USA, see Björkman (1989) and Gaumer (1984) – the latter reviews all the earlier literature. Levin (1980) contains 18 contributions on the regulation of health care but, notably, none directly on the regulation of the medical profession. There are useful chapters on medical education, and on the political environment of regulation. Haug (1976), who studied the USA, UK and USSR, and McKinlay and Arches (1985) both see doctors as in decline, faced with more assertive and demanding states and patients.

On the UK the best general analysis is Klein (1989). Elston (1991) examines the 'proletarianization' thesis advanced in the USA by McKinlay and Arches (1985) and finds it wanting.

On Germany both Altenstetter (1989) and Döhler (1989) link evidence of the German medical profession to the general debate about medical power. For readers of German, the best starting points are Bauch (1982) and Butterfass (1986).

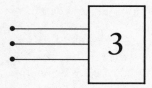

3

THE DEVELOPMENT OF REGULATION

INTRODUCTION

The history of the regulation of doctors is highly varied. The four tasks of regulation identified in Chapter 2 – market entry, competitive practices, market structures and pay – were tackled at different times and in different ways within each country. Yet some common patterns are observable, and before we turn to the detail it is worth noting the most significant.

Perhaps the most important common pattern is that some regulation of doctors always preceded the development of modern health-care systems. The introduction of national insurance in Germany and the UK, of the later UK National Health Service, and of government Medicare and Medicaid programmes in the USA, all raised new issues and required modifications to the existing regulatory structure.

Regulation not only preceded modern health-care systems, it in fact preceded modern health care. Doctors were licensed, for example, before medicine became scientific and before hospitals became places in which people were cured. Doctors were solo practitioners who offered solace and comfort more than diagnosis and treatment. The concept of a profession and of professional regulation came later.

In those early days of solo practitioners medicine was delivered through markets dominated by individual transactions between physician and patient. Services were freely purchased by patients without the intrusion of government health-care programmes, of big complex institutions like modern hospitals, or of the activities of the suppliers of drugs and medical equipment. Licensing was sought by doctors because it could be used to reduce supply and thereby lessen competition and enhance income. Not that this was the line of argument they adopted – rather, the need to protect the public from bad doctors was stressed. The great political skill of eighteenth and early nineteenth century doctors lay in the way in which they managed to convince society that they worked for the public good. Their successors have arguably been equally successful in perpetuating the image: 'the medical profession has benefited from a widespread cultural acceptance of its own self-description as a group of people who serve the public interest' (Stone, 1980a).

A second general feature to emerge from an examination of the historical development of regulation concerns, not the common pattern of experience, but the individual distinctiveness of national attitudes. Take the example of the role of competition in the lives of medical professionals. American culture is one of competitive individualism. This eschews monopolies and has led to demands for governmental intervention against anti-competitive medical practices, like restrictions on advertising. What is known as the Anti-Trust Laws, which were originally designed to prevent commercial or business monopolies, have been much used against the professions, particularly the medical profession, in recent decades. In contrast, in the UK until very recently there have been few government moves to make medicine more competitive. In broad terms, the Europeans were less enamoured of competitive capitalism after the Industrial Revolution and preferred to concentrate on the hierarchical organization of services rather than on cash transfers. Their greater faith in state power over service delivery also led to a more overt level of direct state regulation.

The historical paths of regulation, then, are important in helping to explain the nature, style and extent of contemporary regulation. In this chapter we will first see how the regulation of doctors developed in each of the three main countries of the study, focusing on the balance between the three broad ways of organizing regulation outlined in Chapter 2 (independent self-regulation; state-licensed self-regulation; direct state regulation). The chapter will conclude with an assessment of the extent to which market entry, competitive practices, market structures and pay have in practice been regulated in the past.

REGULATING UK DOCTORS

UK doctors were organized early. The Royal College of Physicians was chartered in the sixteenth century (in 1518), and the College of Surgeons (later the Royal College) separated from the Company of Barbers in 1745. The less well-off relied on the forerunners of today's general practitioners, who were organized into the Society of Apothecaries (Allsop, 1984, pp. 18–23). Each organization constituted a separate self-regulatory body, controlling membership. With medical education and qualifications effectively non-existent, surgeons and physicians in particular were recruited to their organizations more through word of mouth and status than through the display of expertise. Physicians had the highest social status and dominated the supply of medical services, with surgeons in competition.

The collective provision of public health services became essential as the consequences of industrial and urban growth led to water- and sewage-based diseases. Leaders of the public health movement had little time for doctors. Chadwick, the great nineteenth century health-care reformer, spoke of their 'bumbling pretensions' and was critical of the disputes between physicians, surgeons and apothecaries. Many of the latter became parish medical officers under the Poor Law 1834 reforms and, later, District Medical Officers of Health. In a separate development medical directories began to be published in the early 1850s in an attempt by the three branches to clamp down on the thousands of 'doctors' who lacked qualifications (30 000 declared themselves to be doctors in the 1841 Census but only 11 000 appeared in the approved directories).

In terms of taking direct responsibility for services, Parliament restricted its activities to public health and passed a series of acts which initially enabled and later forced local governments to take action. Indirectly it sought to tackle the fragmentation of the medical profession and the inadequacy of medical education and qualifications by establishing a statutory regulatory body under the Medical Act 1858.

Today known as the GMC, or General Medical Council, the new body had the more cumbersome original title General Council of Medical Education and Registration of the United Kingdom. As this suggests, there were two tasks delegated to it – the licensing of individual doctors and the approval of medical schools. Some kind of unity was thus imposed on the fragmented profession, since the registered doctors' list was to include surgeons, physicians, other newer specialists and general practitioners. It still does, with specialist qualifications being determined elsewhere, by the Royal Colleges.

Though statutorily created, the GMC was – and remains – a prime example of state-licensed self-regulation. The 1858 Act – and the several later amending Acts – was a contract between the state and the profession, delegating to the latter responsibility for the standards and quality of those who practise as doctors, a form of contract which UK government has several times utilized to make arrangements with other professions such as law or engineering. Thus the GMC was initially composed solely of doctors appointed by the main professional societies and academic institutions. Today doctors continue to dominate it, accounting for more than 85 per cent of its members, but many are now elected by the profession at large.

The historical significance of the GMC is twofold. First, unlike some countries where direct regulation by the state prevails, in the UK a tradition of a government–profession contract creating a legal regulatory body and hence legitimizing self-regulation was, and still is, the preferred approach. Certainly the privilege of self-regulation has for many decades been much cherished by the UK medical profession. This formal legitimacy makes the GMC that much more authoritative than would be a non-statutory body. This, in turn, connects to the second aspect of historical significance. State-licensed self-regulation is not the same as independent self-regulation in one important respect. Independent self-regulation would be undertaken by the same body that acts as the doctors' trade union – in the UK, the British Medical Association (BMA). Such a body is clearly partisan, having been established primarily to look after the interests of its members. By divorcing regulation from unionism, the 1858 Act actually strengthened the authority of the profession and the GMC, and gave allopathic medicine enormous prestige and status.

Unionism as direct self-regulation still had its part to play. Indeed, a feature of UK medical history is the complexity of regulatory arrangements. Initially responsibility was shared between the GMC and the BMA, with the specialist societies such as the Royal College of Physicians adding to the tangle by approving specialist qualifications. Later, in the twentieth century, more state-created bodies were established following the introduction of national insurance in 1911 and the NHS in 1948 – bodies such as the 1911 Local Insurance Committees which presided over services for the poor through their 'panel' doctors, and the 1948 Medical Practices Committee (all doctors, so an example of state licensed self-regulation) which still presides over the geographical dispersal of general practitioners to ensure that their services are available in approximately equal numbers everywhere.

The BMA, dating from 1855 when it took over from the Provincial Medical and Surgical Association originally founded in 1832, initially primarily represented general practitioners (or apothecaries), the poor relations of the profession. Today it is widely seen as being the leading spokesman for all doctors. It remains an important regulatory body as well as a major negotiator on medical pay. It played a particularly crucial role in resolving intra-profession demarcation disputes in the 1880s: the outcome in effect stamped on the UK the predominant form of medical practice which remains today and which all subsequent governments have accepted when designing national insurance and national health systems – the gatekeeper role of GPs, and the clear division of labour between GPs and hospital doctors through the referral system.

The unity imposed on the profession by the 1858 Act and GMC licensing system was more apparent than real. In practice, jealousies between physicians, surgeons and GPs remained. Indeed, they grew following scientific developments such as antiseptic surgery, the emergence of new specialisms alongside physicians and surgeons, and the increasing importance of hospitals as curative institutions in the second half of the nineteenth century. By the 1880s GP resentment of their higher status hospital colleagues threatened 'a really ugly internecine feud' (Gould, 1985, p. 73) which was resolved through talks between the BMA and the Royal Colleges. The immediate issue was the alleged poaching of patients by the hospital specialists and an agreement was struck whereby these specialists would only see patients referred to them by GPs for a second opinion (thus the title accorded to them of 'consultant'). Hence today's division of labour which forbids direct patient access to specialists, in contrast to the situation in many other countries.

The legacy of history in the UK is now quite clear. The medical profession determined its own boundaries through the state-approved GMC's licensing qualifications (osteopaths, for example, are not accepted for registration as doctors). It negotiated internally a system of patient referral which has become accepted as the way in which medical services should be organized. It established its own codes of conduct through the several Medical Acts which empowered the GMC to determine doctor behaviour and to discipline miscreants. Finally, it developed a strong, more united BMA to act as its spokesman in its relations with government. This was a critical development, because since the founding of the National Health Service in 1948, government has been the monopoly payer for health care, and hence the single key organization with which doctors have to work. Given the high status and functional autonomy of the profession, the existence of government as the sole body with which to negotiate has arguably strengthened its hand.

REGULATING US PHYSICIANS

As in the UK, there was limited respect for doctors in mid-nineteenth century America. Starr (1982) describes them in the 1860s as 'the most despised of the professions'. They lacked the UK guilds or specialist colleges. They lacked control over entry due to the abandonment of state government licensing powers in the 1830s. They lacked social standing and authority. Most medical schools sought only to make money, and offered rudimentary training which might last for no more than a month or two.

In contrast to the UK, the achievement of professional recognition and legitimacy did not get fully under way until the turn of the twentieth century. True, licensing was re-introduced in most states in the 1870s and 1880s, and the state boards were dominated by state governor-appointed doctors who represented the local medical elites. But control over medical education and professional standards had to await the 1903 reforms of the American Medical Association which turned that body into a powerful self-regulatory body as well as an influential spokesman for the profession.

Nineteenth-century US medicine was characterized by division and sectarian dispute. US doctors were not able to fix the boundaries of the profession. Eclectics and homeopaths and, later, osteopaths and chiropractors sought equal status. Orthodox physicians threatened by such sects – those just below the medical élite – most wanted the introduction of examinations and registers, and they were behind the establishment of the American Medical Association in 1847. Their aim was to control supply through controlling medical education, and at the first meeting of the AMA a Committee on Medical Education was appointed.

For more than half a century the AMA failed in its basic aim. It quickly found that many of its own members had a conflict of interests, being owners of, or recipients of fees from, the very medical schools which AMA leaders so despised. Though it took an ostensibly hard line against the alternative sects, the lack of professional standing and legitimacy of doctors meant that the two sides 'fought to a draw' (Starr, 1982, p. 100). Historically the legacy is one of an acceptance in 1903 by the AMA of osteopathy, and a greater tolerance of the existence of chiropractors than in the UK.

Effective regulation through a hierarchy of county and state medical societies and through positive action to control medical education had to wait until the early years of this century. The re-introduction of state board licensing had had little impact on supply because in many states there were, in effect, no meaningful qualifications. The AMA's 8000 members represented only about 7 per cent of doctors in 1900. By 1910 it represented 50 per cent and by 1920 some 60 per cent of doctors following the integration of its organization with the county and state medical societies which controlled the state licensing boards, and which required membership from all doctors who wished to be able to admit patients to hospitals (a form of state-approved self-regulation using the trade union 'closed shop' principle).

Controlling supply took a little longer. The new (1904) AMA Council on Medical Education 'failed' about half the medical schools it inspected, and this led to the Carnegie Foundation-funded Flexner Report of 1910 with its proposals for a dramatic reduction in the numbers of medical schools. The influence of Flexner is debatable – one interpretation is that the demands of state licensing boards for better qualifications and the proven worth of the reformed and new university medical schools, such as Harvard and Johns Hopkins, were already putting the inferior schools out of business. Not in question is that the combination of all these factors led to a fall in the numbers of recognized doctors after 1900.

The AMA's power as a self-regulatory body continued to grow. In 1912 the newly created Federation of State Medical Boards accepted as authoritative the AMAs rating of medical schools. By then its Council on Pharmacy and Chemistry had become a more important regulator of the pharmaceutical industry than the federal regulatory agencies. However, the growth of specialties proved more difficult to regulate, and separate specialty boards outside the AMA became more influential. And hospital standards were accredited following initiatives by the American College of Surgeons within a few years of its 1912 establishment.

The historical legacy of all this activity early in the century is one of predominantly self-regulation, but through complex institutions. State licensing boards which are, in effect, commonly controlled by doctors are comparatively simple in design. Though they may license other health professions as well as doctors, this strengthens the medical profession's position. Doctors, in effect, determine the work of, and qualifications for entry into, several paramedical and therapy professions.

State licensing boards apart, the relative absence of governmental involvement in the history of doctor regulation is in striking contrast to the UK experience of statutorily sanctioned medical schools and occupational licensure. Indeed, the AMA consistently fought to prevent federal involvement, playing on the traditional antipathy of Americans towards government. Until the 1960s it successfully opposed federal funding of medical education. In so doing it kept medical schools few in number so successfully that a chronic shortage of US-trained doctors became apparent in the 1950s, and the large-scale immigration of foreign medical graduates became a necessity. A 1959 government report estimated the need to increase medical student numbers by 50 per cent in order to maintain the doctor: patient ratio, and in 1963 federal funding of medical education began in earnest.

The AMA's opposition to government health-care programmes also held until the 1960s, when Medicare and Medicaid were inaugurated in 1965. The AMA had been concerned about the traditional self-employed status of doctors, with payment being made on a fee-for-service basis, and was bitterly opposed to salaried status or to governmentally determined fee schedules. The Johnson Administration in effect bought off much of the medical opposition by agreeing not to regulate pay but to allow doctors to send in accounts for Medicare patients based on 'usual, customary and prevailing fees'. Another concession allowed the patient to be billed separately for part of the cost, if the Government would not meet it all.

The proposed AMA boycott of the new schemes fizzled out when doctors realized that they were suddenly to be in receipt of millions of extra patients and a virtually guaranteed income increase! (In the UK the post-war Labour Government had used similar types of concession to buy off medical opposition to the NHS – hospital consultants could earn additional income from private treatment and GPs retained their self-employed status.)

Up until the 1970s and 1980s, then, federal government involvement in the regulation of doctors was minimal, and states largely restricted them-selves to licensure. Independent self-regulation only came under pressure when the combination of worldwide economic recession and spiralling health-care costs appeared in the 1970s.

REGULATING GERMAN DOCTORS

The history of the medical profession in Germany, like that of every other important group and institution in the country, has been marked by Germany's own special history, which has been considerably more turbulent than that of the USA or the UK. In the first half of this century alone, for instance, Germany saw the collapse of a monarchy at the end of the First World War; the unstable Weimar Republic which succeeded the monarchy, and which was in turn replaced in 1933 by a Nazi dictatorship under Hitler; the collapse in turn of that dictatorship following Germany's defeat at the end of the Second World War in 1945; and then a period of foreign occupation which was followed by the division of the country at the end of the 1940s into two separate states. These cataclysmic events have all left their mark on the medical profession, and have given it a history which is very different from that of doctors in the more peaceful Anglo-Saxon states. But while German history is distinctive, many of the issues that have concerned the medical profession – control over entry, pay and working conditions – are exactly the same as have concerned US and UK doctors. And although the great turning points in recent German history have left their mark on the medical profession, it is also remarkable how far similar attitudes and institutions have persisted.

The history of doctors in Germany can be divided into four periods: the years before the establishment of the compulsory insurance system in 1883 (the details of which were given in Chapter 2); the period up to the Great Depression at the end of the 1920s; the years until the collapse of Nazi rule in 1945; and the post-war period.

In 1883 Germany had only existed as a unified state for 13 years, and much of the early history of the profession is therefore part of the histories of the states and principalities that preceded the unified German Reich. But though these histories were very different the profession confronted one overwhelming problem which, in essence, was the same as that faced by UK and US doctors in the nineteenth century. This was the question of the occupational status of doctors and, in particular, their position as a 'profession'. The struggle for professional status was critical in the USA and the UK, as we have seen, but it had a particular significance in territories that eventually made up Germany. Professional *status* was precisely that – a distinct legal status marked by particular institutions and by the possession of legally endowed rights and duties. A key distinction existed between occupations considered to be businesses engaged in trade, and publicly regulated as such, and those allowed the status of regulating themselves through their own chamber, a public law body granted legal powers and duties by the state (Stone, 1980, p. 36ff).

Designation as the latter gave exemptions from codes governing trade; allowed the occupation to establish in the 'chamber' a body whose membership was compulsory for those practising the occupation; and this compulsory membership in turn allowed chambers the right to represent the occupation and control occupational practices. Organization into a 'chamber' with public law status was a common pattern. Thus, what doctors struggled to achieve was a legal position in no way unique; it was the recognized badge that separated a professional occupation from the conventional activities of competitive business.

Possession of this prized status was only slowly achieved in Germany. At unification in 1870 only some of the component states who made up the new Reich had allowed their doctors to set up chambers, and despite physicians' lobbying no German-wide law mandating 'chamber' status was established after 1870. Although several of the constituent parts of the new German state did eventually permit doctors to form self-governing chambers (Prussia, for instance, in 1887) it was not until 1935, under the Nazis, that an all-German code established that medicine was a profession distinctive from trade and entitled to regulate itself through public law chambers. This 1935 code is the basis of the present legal status of doctors in Germany as a free profession.

By the 1930s, however, the politics of regulation in Germany had been deeply influenced by the consequences of the health insurance reforms of 1883. These reforms introduced into health-care a set of institutions – the health insurance funds – which for over 50 years were to have an uneasy and often conflicting relationship with doctors.

Part of the reason for this relationship of conflict lay in the contrasting political aims of the funds and doctors. At heart, the majority of doctors – who were in 'solo' practice – were involved in small business; insurance funds, until the 1930s, were closely tied to the trade unions and the left-wing political parties. These political differences, however, only magnified an even more important source of conflict: the health insurance reforms of 1883 drastically altered the nature of the market in the services of doctors. Initially the funds covered only a small proportion of the population, and chiefly existed to provide insurance cover for loss of earnings due to sickness. But in the two decades after the passing of the original law their role and importance changed greatly. Their membership grew, from 4.29 million in 1885 to 13.36 million in 1911. Their responsibilities expanded from providing insurance for loss of income to actually paying for treatment. In other words, they became major contributors to the salaries of doctors. Until the beginning of the 1930s medical politics were dominated by the attempts of the profession to minimize the control which this fact gave the funds over doctors. The conflict was intensified because many of the funds were direct employers of doctors: some organized their own medical services, taking on doctors as paid employees; in other cases doctors, though they were in free practice, were tied contractually to a fund. All this undermined the aspirations of doctors to the status of a 'free profession'. The conflict was made more intense still, especially in the period after the First World War, by the oversupply of doctors, which depressed physician income.

This phase in the history of the profession was marked by the gradual emergence among doctors of organizations to counteract the power of the health insurance funds. There took place in the early decades of the century a set of bitter conflicts. A series of compromises gave the doctors some increased independence from the funds, but still, at the end of the 1920s, left the funds with significant control over the working practices of physicians.

The events of the third important historical phase – covering the first half of the 1930s – decisively changed the balance of advantage in favour of the medical profession. The turning point happened outside medicine. After 1929 Germany, like most other western countries, suffered a great economic collapse as the world economy entered the Great Depression. In Germany the crisis was particularly severe. In 1930 and 1931 this crisis forced Government intervention in the health-care system, chiefly in order to cut the cost of insurance contributions and to limit benefits. The upshot was significantly to curtail the freedom of the doctors' main rivals – the insurance funds – freely to offer services and to set their own contribution and benefit levels. But from the doctors' point of view the most important change lay in the fact that in reforms introduced in 1931 they wrested from the funds the power to pay individual doctors for the treatment of patients – and it had been the fact that funds could act as the direct paymasters of doctors which was seen as the greatest threat to physicians' status as free professionals. The reforms created new associations of insurance doctors, membership of which was compulsory for those doctors who treated patients from the funds. (By this period over half the population was covered by the insurance system.) These associations of insurance doctors were public law bodies who took over from the insurance funds key responsibilities for the provision of medical care outside hospitals: they had the duty of ensuring that doctors were available to provide care; they could regulate its quality and cost; they acted as the contractor with individual doctors; and they negotiated a lump sum payment from the insurance funds for the total cost of treatment, paying individual doctors from that lump sum. In short, these reforms marked a great increase in the control exercised by doctors over their own working conditions, and repulsed the most significant threat to their position as free professionals engaged in solo practice.

These reforms were the start of a period when doctors advanced to establish their professional independence, and to become the dominant group in the health-care system. After the Nazi seizure of power the doctors' chief rivals, the insurance funds, suffered great persecution because of their connections with trade unionism and socialism. By contrast, doctors were among the most enthusiastic supporters of the Nazis – a support rewarded with the grant of national status as a free profession in 1935.

This third period was dramatically ended with the defeat of Germany and the collapse of the Nazi regime in 1945. The close identification of the medical profession with the Nazis, coupled with the collapse of the whole Nazi system, might have been expected to damage the independence and prestige which doctors had gained in the reforms of the 1930s. Indeed, in the Eastern Zone, which in 1949 became the Soviet Union-sponsored German Democratic Republic, doctors were tightly controlled by the state and were, by Western standards, poorly paid. But the striking feature of the larger and more prosperous Federal Republic which emerged in the rest of Germany was the extent to which the patterns of the 1930s soon reasserted themselves.

Immediately after the War an attempt was made, with the support of left wing politicians, to persuade the Occupying Powers to replace the old multiplicity of insurance funds with a single, nationwide, publicly controlled health insurance fund, but this was soon abandoned. By the time the Federal Republic was established in 1949 the old system of a multiplicity of funds had begun to be re-established. In the next six years the new German Government restored most of what had been established in the 1930s. This meant that doctors once more emerged as the dominant group in the health-care system. The 'chambers' for the profession existing in the Nazi period had been dissolved by the Allies immediately after the War, but as early as 1947 new chambers to regulate the profession began to be re-established in individual states, like Bavaria.

The decade after 1945 saw a struggle, largely successful, on the part of doctors to ensure that the insurance funds were not allowed to resume their historical role as employers of doctors or as direct providers of medical services. The doctors' victory was sealed by the reforms of 1955, which cast the health-care system into its present mould. The health insurance funds and the associations of insurance doctors were confirmed as public law organizations. The functions assumed by the insurance doctors' associations in the reforms introduced in the early 1930s, were explicitly restored to them: they acquired the duty to ensure that doctoring services were available outside hospitals, and to inspect the doctors who provided those services; they were to negotiate with the insurance funds over the payment for these services; and, using the revenue received from the services, they were to meet the claims of individual doctors for payment. By the middle of the 1950s, in other words, the insurance funds were once again clearly restricted to raising the resources to pay for care; the doctors had restored their status as free professionals, largely operating in solo practices, and contracted only to their own associations.

By the mid-1950s, the modern system of regulation in Germany had been established. It was a system in which doctors occupied once again a dominant position. Much has happened in the intervening years – partly to strengthen, and partly to weaken, the position of doctors. But it is from the mid-1950s that the present system recognizably dates, and it is an appropriate moment to end this historical sketch.

HISTORICAL PATTERNS IN REGULATION

Historical patterns of regulation show different emphases on self-and state-regulation, and different timescales in each of our three countries. In addition, the amount of regulation varied. In this section each of the four tasks of regulation outlined in Chapter 2, will be examined.

Market entry

The issue of who can qualify for recognition as a doctor was handled very differently, as the examples of the UK and the USA show. UK divisions were largely *within* the medical profession, and were regulated by demarcation agreements over the boundaries and roles of specialists and of general practitioners, made in the 1880s by the BMA and the specialist colleges and still the basis of medical organization today. Much earlier the Medical Act 1858 had, in effect, legalized the monopoly of 'orthodox' medicine and driven away claimants to the title of doctor who lacked qualifications. This medical monopoly has since been used to deny the claims of osteopaths, chiropractors, and homeopathic practitioners, among others, to be accepted as medical practitioners. State-sanctioned self-regulation led to early tight control of the definition of 'doctor' and of 'medicine'.

The US experience was more of divisions *between* orthodox medicine and sects. US doctors lacked 'the esoteric learning, knowledge of Latin, and high culture and status of traditional English physicians' (Starr, 1982, p. 17), and consequently lacked authority. In addition, what licensing they had (which anyway was ineffective) disappeared in the 1830s and 1840s under Jacksonian ideology. This lack of authority, power and legitimacy prevented them from establishing English-type professional boundaries until early in the twentieth century, and even then the medical lobby was unable to prevent the licensure of osteopathy and of chiropractors in nearly every state 'despite vehement medical opposition' (Starr, 1982, p. 126). On the other hand, this opposition had some successes in denying such alternative treaters the rights of access to hospitals and of prescribing drugs. Hence though alternative therapies have had to be accepted, orthodox medicine eventually climbed into the driving seat after a nineteenth century era of only equal status with the sects.

Market entry affects supply, and every profession has a clear interest in controlling supply so as to prevent a surplus. Again, the UK profession scored an early success through the legislative creation of the GMC: at a stroke, as it were, some 60 per cent of those who claimed to be a doctor disappeared. The number and size of medical schools and the immigration regulations are other crucial factors. In the UK both have been the preserve of governments since the Second World War, using the General Medical Council machinery to monitor foreign medical graduates, and the university funding institutions to give financial support to medical schools.

The American profession had much greater regulatory control over both medical schools (after the Flexner Report of 1910) and foreign medical graduates. US medical students and schools did not receive large government grants, unlike the British. The medical profession was able to lay down standards, and to drive out the plethora of rudimentary medical schools which had not come to terms with the development of the science of medicine (some even lacked any laboratory accommodation, for example). So successful was it that by the 1950s there was an acute shortage of doctors. The regulatory intervention of the federal government in 1963 has, by the 1990s, led to the opposite scenario of oversupply and of a reluctance of taxpayer-supported medical schools to cut intakes.

The most striking feature of the German experience has been the way influences largely external to the health-care system itself have so often influenced the supply of doctors – usually by threatening an over-supply. The most recurrent of these is the higher education system itself, where a historically embedded tradition of open admission to university courses for all formally qualified applicants has been the dominant influence in medical education. A second notable feature is the way the cataclysmic history of Germany has so often administered a shock to the 'supply' system: the end of both the First and Second World Wars, for instance, produced a doctor surplus, through demobilization of armed forces and movements of population. What the German historical experience emphasizes is that there is no uniform historical route of professional regulation; the details of a country's history matter greatly.

Competitive practices

As professionals, doctors eschew normal commercial practices designed to increase trade. They claim to value 'consumer protection', and to work solely in 'the public interest'. When translated, such phrases mean that doctors are the best people to determine the needs of their patients. They also mean that colleagues should not interfere in the doctor–patient relationship unless and until the outcome of that relationship is a call for a second opinion. A 'bedside monopoly' is thus created, allegedly to the benefit of the patient and certainly to the benefit of the doctor.

Historically the Medical Act 1858 might have challenged some of these tenets in the UK. The new GMC was to create one register containing all doctors' names and not differentiating whether they were physicians, surgeons or general practitioners. However, this state-created self-regulatory body was able to lay down ethical codes of conduct which had, and have, to be satisfied if a doctor is to remain licensed. Such codes have always included rules about unprofessional behaviour which are designed to prevent or minimize competition. In the 1970 GMC booklet, for example, the 'largest emphasis is placed on those crimes which could interfere with trade' (Gould, 1985, p. 101). Twelve column inches were devoted to advertising and not to criticizing a competitor, with less than two inches each to neglect of a patient and misuse of dangerous drugs.

Probably more significant historically was the self-regulated agreement reached in the 1880s over referrals and the GP gatekeeper role. This effectively abolished direct access for patients to hospital specialists and established the codified or regulated notion of intra-professional demarcation. Subsequently the professional bodies have built on this precedent and have laid down guidelines about the boundaries between physicians and psychiatrists, orthopaedic surgeons and radiologists, and so on. The sub-specialties of UK medicine have a history of being very sharply defined.

Much of this is in direct contrast with recent US experience, and some of it with the American tradition. US doctors followed the UK approach and agreed to a 'no commercialism' code of conduct, which held sway until the successful attempt by government in the 1970s and 1980s to apply federal Anti-Trust Laws to the professions. The supreme court upheld those laws and outlawed such activities as bans on advertising and boycotts to undermine new health-care delivery systems based on capitation payments rather than on fee-for-service. These systems had been initiated with the active support of the federal government as they were expected to reduce health-care expenditure.

On the other hand, the American tradition never embraced the concept of the general practitioner as a gatekeeper. Instead the USA retained 'fluid boundaries within the profession' (Starr, 1982, p. 225). Patients had, and have, direct access to specialists, and GPs retained admitting rights at hospitals because the new specialty boards lacked any powers to insist that hospitals only employed their members. In the long run, however, such powers were not needed. As medicine became more and more specialized the demise of the GP, except in rural areas, became inevitable.

In the German case, the historical struggle over competition was centred on the attempts by the doctors to secure recognition from the state as a profession, by requiring 'chamber' status. As we saw earlier, this came relatively late, with the granting of such a status nationwide in the Nazi period of the 1930s.

Market structures

Moves to regulate the freedom of licensed doctors to set up in practice wherever they want were rare in both the UK and USA until the post-War period. Self-regulated ethical codes about advertising restricted the amount of overt competition in both countries, but had little or no impact on the geographical distribution of doctors.

In the USA, the perceived market for services continues to determine practice location. Consequently there are enormous differences in the availability of medical services. As we have mentioned previously, attractive and affluent cities can have as few as 176 patients per doctor (as in the case of San Francisco). Poorer rural areas have more than 3500 patients per doctor and in 1985 as many as 13.5 million Americans lived in such underserved areas. The only general regulatory response has been to use the inducement of student scholarships, awarded on condition that the recipients would work for 2–4 years in such areas. Begun in 1972, this scheme of National Health Service Corps Physicians was wound up by the Reagan Administration in the mid-1980s. In any event its impact was offset by the simultaneous decline in family practice, and the improved spread of doctors in the last 20 years owes more to the general increase in numbers than to any regulatory action aimed at geographic distribution.

The UK, too, had a strikingly inequitable geographic distribution of doctors until well into the twentieth century – again because the market rather than regulation determined location. This remains true for dentists, where there are twice as many per capita in the south as in the north of England. But there have been state-led restrictions on doctors since 1948. At the hospital level this has been through budgetary control, with hospital managers having fixed allocations which, in effect, limit their medical complements. Though doctors have been influential advisers at ministry, hospital and regional health authority levels, this can scarcely be described as self-regulation. Ensuring an equitable distribution of self-employed general practitioners has, however, been achieved through state-led self-regulation: the national Medical Practices Committee authorizes applications from doctors to set up in practice using a strict doctor:population ratio to determine whether or not a town or district is 'open', 'restricted' or 'closed'.

Group practice and salaried status have historically caused greater concern to the American self-regulators than to their British equivalents. For a century or more, the American Medical Association fiercely opposed the latter as leading to cut-price care and as threatening the doctor–patient relationship which was based entirely on patient needs and not on the interests of a doctor's employer. The AMA was also concerned about group practices when they first become fashionable, and regularly pointed to the dangers of doctors becoming, in effect, corporations.

Eventually the AMA had to modify its outright opposition to salaried status as the practice spread in larger hospitals and, later, in the community with the 1970s growth of Health Maintenance Organizations (HMOs). In the UK, in contrast, the salaried status of hospital doctors has not been a major issue. The 1880s division of labour agreement confirmed a clear distinction between hospital and general practice medicine. In later negotiations (in 1946–8) doctors struck a deal with the Government enabling them to add to their salaries through private work.

In Germany, the historical struggles over market structures were, we have seen, decisively resolved after the Nazi seizure of power – because with that seizure the insurance funds were destroyed as providers of health care and as employers of doctors.

Payment regulation

US doctors (with some exceptions, as in the case of HMOs) set their own fee levels. These vary considerably, from area to area and between doctors in the same area. Historically the only restrictions have been any imposed by a patient (which is unlikely, for most patients have no idea of the 'going rate' for anything more than a routine appointment fee), by an insurance company, or by government. Widespread health insurance is a relatively recent phenomenon, beginning in the 1930s but only really developing in the 1945–60 period. By then the medical profession had become very powerful and its authority and legitimacy, coupled with patients' dependence on it, made challenging fee levels difficult, even for large insurance companies. In any event, in that period cost containment was not an issue – so much so that the federal government, too, was happy to negotiate doctor-determined fees for Medicare and Medicaid patients in 1965. It was the cost explosion which followed that caused fee regulation to become a policy issue.

In the UK, fee regulation at the general practice level has a much longer history. Local Insurance Committees paid doctors for treating 'panel' patients from 1911, and by the time the NHS was established in 1948 the concept of government-determined fee schedules, published only after negotiation of a closed, corporatist nature, was accepted by doctors. An important consequence of this and of the GP–hospital division with salaried hospital doctors has been that UK doctors have only a limited incentive to treat patients. In contrast, US doctors, whose incomes are determined by their levels of activity, have every incentive to treat patients. The outcomes of these distinctive historical approaches to pay regulation are striking. American patients are three times more likely to have surgery, and are subjected to many more diagnostic tests than are the British. At the national level, the USA spends almost 12 per cent of its Gross National Product on health care; the UK spends only 6 per cent.

The 1948 NHS settlement of pay systems was acceptable in principle to all, with its corporatist negotiating machinery led by the BMA. But within a decade doctors had become sufficiently dissatisfied with negotiating direct with government that they obtained an inquiry by a Royal Commission into their pay. In 1960 the Pilkington Commission concluded in favour of an independent review body to recommend the remuneration of doctors and dentists, and this now annually receives evidence from both the professions and government.

Government is pledged to accept the Remuneration Board's findings, though it has sometimes delayed or phased in full implementation. The Remuneration Board has not examined one substantial 'perk' negotiated in 1948 – the system of 'Merit Awards' for hospital consultants. About one-third of consultants are in receipt of such an award, payable at one of three levels and amounting to over £6000 per annum (or 14 per cent of basic salary) at the lowest level. The profession has determined the recipients, and the process is very secret. It remains a curious legacy of history, an example of buying out opposition which, after four decades, has become institutionalized and difficult to remove or radically change.

In Germany the critical historical episodes occurred, as often in other areas of medical regulation, in the early 1930s. It was then, with the foundation of the Insurance Doctors' Associations, that payment regulation in the dominant part of the profession, local practice, took on its present form: collective bargaining for a global sum between payers (the insurance funds) and the doctors' associations, with the latter controlling payment to individual physicians.

CONCLUSION

Three themes emerge with particular clarity from these historical sketches. The first is the universal aspiration of doctors for professional status: by which they have meant self-regulation, and the use of the institutions of regulation to restrict competition and impose common standards. Second, in all three countries, the development of doctors as professionals has interacted with two other features of the health-care system: the rise of modern medicine, with its scientific base, its numerous specialisms and its developing relations with a host of ancillary medical occupations; and the rise of government as a major institution in the organization of health care.

These two themes stress the common experiences of doctors. But a third feature to emerge clearly from these pages emphasizes something which will recur as our discussion unfolds – the uniqueness of national experience. Doctors have some aspirations in common, and face some common pressures. But these aspirations and pressures have been mediated, not just by the particular history of national professions, but by the wider national history. It is true of all our three cases, but it emerges with particular clarity in the German case, where the history of the medical profession is inseparable from the milestones in the nation's development – unification, world wars, dictatorship, division and, lastly, at the end of the 1980s, re-unification. Germany stands as an illustration of our wider theme: the tension between national uniqueness and common professional aspirations and pressures.

FURTHER READING

There is a brief account of British history in Allsop (1984), pp. 18–23. The General Medical Council's record is examined by Stacey (1989), who traces the rise of, first, elected doctors and, later, lay nominees to membership. The strength of both the GMC and the British Medical Association is heavily criticized by Gould (1985), who describes them in chapter 3 as constituting the core of the 'medical mafia'. An equally swingeing attack on the US profession is in Inlander *et al.* (1988). A more sober assessment of the limitations of curative medicine is in McKeown (1980).

The early efforts of US physicians to organize themselves into an effective, protective political force are comprehensively charted in chapters 1–3 of Starr (1982). Ludmerer (1985) concentrates on the history of US medical schools, including the impact of the Flexner Report of 1910. In chapter 6, Starr (1982) goes on to describe the generally successful boycotting by US doctors of any attempts to employ them on a salaried basis at the workplace, an issue also examined by Walsh (1987). Ebert in chapter 5 of Schramm (1987) reviews the AMA's successful attempts early in the century to remove rivals. Colombotos and Kirchner (1986) see the conservative AMA as under pressure from an increasingly liberal profession at the grass roots.

Wilsford (1991) explains in chapter 3 the long history of the failure of US governments to enter the health-care arena, and he contrasts this with the French experience.

Marmor and Thomas (1972) review physicians' pay battles in the 1960s in the USA and the UK and conclude that doctors were highly successful in both countries, and in Sweden too. Fox (1987) argues that the period 1911–65 in the USA and UK saw the rise of the hospital as the central institution of medical care, but that this did not remove power from doctors. Freddi (1989) contends that any cross-national comparisons of regulatory history need to take into account different political cultures relating to factors such as competition, individualism, and the role of government. US political ideology is clearly and succinctly set out in relation to the medical profession by Stone (1980a).

Sources for the historical development of the German medical profession in English are scarce. The German section of this chapter draws heavily on Stone (1980b), the pre-eminent text in English. In addition, Rosenberg (1986) is authoritative on the historical development of the insurance funds, and Heidenheimer (1980) compares the historical development of Germany with that in Scandinavia. Jennings (1987) contrasts the rise of the profession in England and the USA with the situation in other European states.

For German readers the key sources are Tennstedt (1977), which is authoritative in the developments from the original health insurance reforms of 1883; and Webber (1988) which reconstructs the history from the crisis caused by the Great Depression. Von Ferber (1989) provides an account of the crucial years of reconstruction after the Second World War.

THE ANATOMY OF REGULATION

INTRODUCTION

We now know that each country has in the past tackled the problems of regulating doctors differently. The balance between self-and state-regulation varies. The style of regulation, and its extent, is peculiar to a particular nation. On the other hand, in Chapter 2 similarities of approach also became apparent. Everywhere there has been debate about the desirable extent of professional autonomy. How far to rely on professions to themselves regulate their members' behaviour has been a common issue. From these debates have emerged a number of alternative regulatory schemes.

Whatever the history, and whatever the outcome of domestic debates about the proper role of doctors, every regulatory scheme in the developed world is based on institutions: in other words, each country has specialized organizations developed for the purpose of regulating doctors. How those institutions work, how effectively and with what results, is the subject of Chapters 5 and 6. But before we look at the dynamics of regulation we must perform a more immediate operation. The actual structure of regulatory institutions needs to be described. That is the purpose of this short chapter.

Institutions are important because their existence alone is a significant determinant of the extent and nature of regulation. Historically, how they came to exist and how they began to operate is also important because this establishes a working method which often continues long after the pioneers have left the scene. Institutional arrangements are part of the culture of medicine in a particular country.

This culture, in turn, is linked to the wider political structure. The UK, for example, has a predominantly centralized political system, usually described as 'unitary' government. In contrast, Germany and the USA have 'federal' constitutions, based on the principle of sharing political power between at least two levels of government, the national and the regional or more local level. In the UK we would, as a result, expect to find national regulatory institutions laying down national rules, even if these are interpreted and applied by local bodies. In Germany and the USA the situation will depend on the outcome of historical processes. Medicine and health care could be seen as either a federal or a local responsibility, or could be a shared or a divided responsibility. A shared responsibility involves institutional arrangements allowing for representation from both the federal or national and the regional or local levels. Divided responsibility means that certain aspects of regulation centre on nationwide institutions, with other aspects being the responsibility of quite separately constituted local bodies.

The task of this chapter is to build on the historical paths of regulation identified in Chapter 3, and to outline the major contemporary regulatory institutions of each of the three countries. These are the institutions which are particularly concerned with the four tasks of regulation examined in Chapter 2 – market entry, competitive practices, market structure and pay. In the next chapter we go on to review the operations of the main institutions as regulators of these key tasks: their processes of decision, formality or informality, and the extent to which they can be described as instances of professional self-regulation or as examples of governmental dominance of the regulatory process.

THE UK'S REGULATORY INSTITUTIONS

We saw in Chapter 3 that UK medicine and politics have a long history of being intermingled. Parliament established the General Medical Council as long ago as 1858. Since 1911 and, more particularly, since the founding of the National Health Service in 1948, Parliament has also taken final responsibility for the financing and delivery of health care. As its name implies, the National Health Service is based on the principle of centralization, even though it is managed and operated locally by appointed boards.

It is, however, important at the outset to distinguish between state control of, and state approval of, regulatory institutions. The National Health

Service, with its fixed budgets and plethora of governmental rules and managerial guidelines, approximates to the common idea of state control (and consequently has long been dubbed by its US critics as 'socialized medicine'). But the regulation of doctors is, in fact, much closer to the idea of state approval than to state control, as the example of the General Medical Council shows.

The General Medical Council (GMC) was the outcome of a mid-nineteenth century bargain which the profession struck with the state and, despite its claim to be there to safeguard patients' interests, it was essentially created to protect doctors, not the public. At a stroke, allopathic medicine became the established or recognized medicine of the UK, with the GMC as the prime advisory body to government on health matters. Parliament's new creation was constituted almost solely of doctors appointed by such institutions as the Royal Colleges (or professional guilds) and the universities with medical schools. It was thus dominated by the leaders of the profession who also had a high social status. Until the 1970s only a handful were doctors elected by their colleagues, and even fewer were non-doctors (the last restricted to three Crown, or government, appointees).

The GMC remains doctor dominated despite two decades of almost unbroken critical debate and the recent introduction of reforming legislation. The criticisms have come from two very different angles. Politicians and consumer groups have sought greater 'lay' or non-medical membership in an attempt to make the GMC less of a closed shop and more accountable to society for its actions. Rank-and-file doctors, on the other hand, have sought more elected medical members on the grounds that the GMC was out of touch with the real world of medical practice. This doctor opposition to the GMC's élitist composition was sparked off primarily by a GMC decision in 1969 to alter the basis of its fees. Until then a doctor, on being admitted to the GMC's approved medical register, paid a life membership fee and could promptly forget about the existence of the GMC as long as he behaved professionally. A shortage of cash (the GMC is self-funding, deriving no finance from general tax resources) caused the Council to introduce a small annual re-registration fee, a policy radical enough to lead the British Medical Association (see below) to call for an immediate rebellion, which was strong enough to result in a government appointed inquiry (the Merrison Committee).

These twin criticisms, by consumers and by doctors, led to statutory changes to the GMC's élite composition in 1979 and 1987. In 1990 of its 102 members a small majority (54) were elected by grass-roots registered doctors. There remain 35 Royal College, university and specialist society appointees, coupled with 13 government nominees. The latter now include 11 who can be described as 'lay' members – though their numbers embrace a nurse and a pharmacist. The remaining nine have varying backgrounds – two Members of Parliament, an accountant, a lawyer, a retired civil servant for example. The one obvious consumer representative is the long-serving leading light of the Patients' Association, a national pressure group.

In terms of membership, the GMC is thus essentially an example of a state-approved self-regulatory professional institution. The recent increase to 11 lay members is of little consequence in a body of over one hundred. Indeed, lay involvement is numerically much less than in the case of other self-regulatory professional institutions created by statute such as the Press Council and the Advertising Standards Authority. As we will see in Chapter 5, GMC powers are considerable. It plays a fundamental part in the admission, behaviour and disciplining of all doctors who practise in the UK.

The GMC does not, however, have a monopoly of regulation. Other key regulatory institutions in the UK are the government (as both the employer of many doctors and the provider of most health care), and the British Medical Association, a pressure group representing doctors' interests, but also an institution playing a central role in regulation.

Though the UK is a unitary state and the NHS a national service, in practice the term 'the government' is a blanket one covering a fragmented set of institutions which make and execute health-care policy. At ministerial level the Department of Health is the leading institution in England. For Wales, Scotland and Northern Ireland there are separate government departments, but they normally take their lead from the Department of Health.

As part of the management reforms of the mid-1980s an attempt was made to separate the Department's role as policy-maker from the day-to-day execution of health policy. The creation of a NHS Management Board to supervise the 300 or so regional and local health authorities was only partly successful. Initially it was to be located outside the Department and its first chief executive was recruited from big business, but it quickly became physically located in the Department's headquarters, headed by a former Regional Health Authority manager, and was renamed the NHS Management Executive.

The Department of Health, like most UK major government departments, has over the years appointed many advisory committees. These have restricted remits and focus on technical issues. Apart from their substantive work they are important in ensuring that there are continual and regular links between government and the medical profession, links which survived the great political explosions such as the doctors' campaigns against the 1948 and the 1989–91 reforms. There is in fact a network of policy-makers in being which essentially spans two camps: the Department, run by civil servants and responsible for the NHS, and the medical profession, represented by both the Royal Colleges and the British Medical Association.

Most of the Royal Colleges (of Surgeons, of Physicians, and so on) date from before the development of an industrial society in the UK, let alone the development of modern health care (though the Royal College of General Practitioners was established only in the 1950s). Prestigious bodies, they focus almost exclusively on clinical issues, promulgating standards of care and respected views on medical ethics. Only occasionally do they behave in an overtly political manner, but their influence on doctors' behaviour is continuous and marked.

The key regulatory institution within the profession as a whole is the British Medical Association. The BMA represents all doctors and negotiates with the Department over all aspects of doctors' activities – pay, conditions of service, and so on – as well as regulating doctors' private work. It has for many years been officially recognized by government as the sole negotiating body on behalf of the medical profession.

The BMA, self-styled the 'champion of social reform' is, in fact and in law, a registered trade union. Its prime aim is thus to further its members' (the doctors) interests. Despite this, it is an integral part of the regulatory structure. It speaks on behalf of all doctors even though its membership was in 1980 only about 50 per cent of registered physicians (there was a sharp increase to around 75 per cent later in the decade following a deliberate campaign to attract 'moderates' by playing down threats of strike action and concentrating more on 'good health' campaigns about issues like smoking and drinking). The Association is accepted as the 'voice of doctors' because, while it has rivals, they are smaller and narrower in their range. The Medical Practitioners Union, for example, has only 4000 members, is affiliated to the Trades Union Congress (the BMA is not), and is thus more overtly 'political'. The BMA had a total membership, home and overseas, of just under 85 000 in 1990.

Under trade union law the BMA has, since 1984, had to adopt a more democratic structure. Only the 46 elected members of its core policy-making body, the BMA Council, now have voting rights on policy issues. But fewer than half of BMA members bother to vote at Council elections.

In addition to the Council, which meets five times a year, the BMA has an annual Representative Meeting of 600 elected doctors and, more important, a whole series of committees with much autonomy and subject to only very limited control from Council. Four have sole negotiating rights on NHS pay – four because the profession is divided into sub-groups covering general practitioners, hospital consultants, public health doctors and hospital juniors. Other BMA committees handle areas such as the impact of the European Community, medicine in the Armed Forces, university doctors, doctors and social work, and private practice.

As a trade union the BMA is, of course, not bound to accept government policy (whereas the GMC, by law, must accept and work within the detailed statutory provisions of Medical Acts). The BMA has a long record of both lobbying government to take action to protect its members (the original Medical Act 1858 was the first example), and of lobbying its members to undermine the implementation of government policy, which can include government-sponsored Acts of Parliament. The threatened boycott of the NHS in 1946–8, after the NHS Act 1946 had been passed, illustrates the attempted use of industrial action. More recently, the BMA at one point pressurized its members to boycott key parts of the government's 1989–91 NHS reforms in an attempt to get the government to modify its plans.

The GMC, Department of Health, Royal Colleges and BMA are the key national regulatory institutions in the UK. Though the Department has its geographical hierarchy of executive health authorities, and the Colleges and BMA have local branches, regulation in the UK is an essentially centralized activity. Health authorities and College and BMA branches are concerned with the local interpretation of national decisions and are thus basically implementors rather than policy makers.

The complete 'real world' is much more complex than the sketch we have presented. The Department of Health, for example, is made up of several dozen 'divisions', and the *BMA Guide* lists its own 28 activity sections, plus no fewer than 49 non-BMA organizations which directly impinge on those activities. The nomenclature can also be misleading due to overlapping acronyms. Thus the GMC is the statutory General Medical Council whilst the GMSC is no more than a sub-group of the BMA – the General Medical Services Committee – which negotiates with the Department of Health on behalf of general practitioners.

US REGULATORY INSTITUTIONS

We saw in Chapter 3 that, historically, the regulation of doctors in the USA was predominantly self-regulation. The dominant regulatory institution has been the American Medical Association, working alongside a number of other professional institutions, including bodies like the Colleges of Surgeons, and of Physicians. The AMA claims to be 'the voice of American medicine', and is recognized as one of the most powerful of all American interest groups, whose support or consent is normally required if any proposed health-care reforms are to have much chance of being implemented. Like the British Medical Association, the AMA is first and foremost a trade union, working to safeguard the interests of its members. However, because of its initiatives in developing self-regulation in the early part of this century, and because of its setting within a political culture which is distrustful of government, the Association has become widely accepted as the appropriate body to regulate doctors in the public interest.

Although an enormous organization, with a staff of over 900, a multi-storey office block headquarters in Chicago, and a sizeable presence in Washington, the AMA in fact can scarcely be said to be fully representative of the US medical profession, because only about 45 per cent of doctors are members. From its historical roots it traditionally has been strongly supportive of the solo family practitioner. This has led to internal tensions as the profession has changed and as specialty groups have grown in strength. Early in the 1970s there was, for example, a struggle before students and interns (junior hospital doctors) achieved representation. Later, in 1977, the AMA was only able to amend its constitution to give greater weight to clinical specialisms after an extremely heated debate lasting several hours.

This greater weight was to be given through changed representation on the AMA's key policy-making body, the House of Delegates. In truth, the AMA was at a low ebb in the 1970s, having lost its fight to prevent the adoption of Medicare and Medicaid, and having overstretched itself financially. Wider representation and a hefty increase in subscriptions were the solutions, but their success was questionable. Membership fell sharply among established doctors, by around 10 per cent in the three years after dues were increased in 1975, though an influx of students and interns masked this. And the increased representation given to specialists upset not only the traditional members but also some of the more prominent specialist groups. The American College of Surgeons, for instance, was dissatisfied with its allocation of only a single member on the House of Delegates to represent the 48 000 surgeons, and refused to take up the place.

As a large policy-making body, the House of Delegates meets only a few times each year. The key executive institution within the AMA is its 17 member Board of Trustees, each of whom is required to devote more than a day a week to the role. Below it are seven councils and dozens of committees which report to the Board, but which have in practice considerable autonomy. The Board of Trustees is essentially a coordinating body, the equivalent of an industrial Board of Directors, headed by a powerful Chairman and overseeing the work of the AMA's senior officials.

The AMA works with many other professional organizations in its regulatory role (in contrast to its political role as a doctors' pressure group, when it may distance itself from, or be distanced by, some of its regulatory partners). Typical examples of inter-organizational cooperation over regulation include arrangements for the accreditation of medical schools (by the Liaison Committee for Medical Education); the licensing of doctors (through examinations by state licensing boards, set by the National Board of Medical Examiners); the accreditation of hospitals; of foreign medical graduates' courses; and of continuing postgraduate training. In each case the regulatory process involves multi-organizational representation on joint regulatory boards, but is in essence independent self-regulation (if sometimes with token non-medical involvement). The 23-member Accreditation Council for Graduate Medical Education, a typical example, is made up of representatives from the following bodies:

American Board of Medical Specialties (4)
AMA (4)
American Hospital Association (4)
Association of American Medical Colleges (4)
Council of Medical Specialty Societies (4)
AMA Resident Physicians Section (1)
Public (1)
Federal Government (1 – non-voting)

Thus far we have examined the AMA at the national (or federal) level. But the strength of the organization after its internal reforms of 1901 was derived from its confederate structure, based on state and local medical societies. For a time these, too, were important regulatory bodies affecting local market structures and competitive behaviour through the exercise of monopoly powers. Today, however, these local regulatory powers have largely disappeared and the membership of local medical societies has fallen rapidly since a 1982 AMA decision that it was no longer obligatory for members to also join a local or state society. Hence the AMA's confederate structure is now rather weak.

It will be plain that one of the most striking features of US regulatory institutions is the central position occupied by what is formally a private pressure group, the American Medical Association. But governmental institutions are also important. The oldest of these are the state licensing boards, the local equivalents of the UK General Medical Council. Under the federal constitution, each of the 50 states has its own Board. The exact titles of the boards differ, as do their composition – though many AMA members are normally on state boards.

In addition, at both state and federal level there are new governmental regulatory institutions following the creation in 1965 of the Medicare and Medicaid programmes. The federal Department of Health and Human Services includes the Health Care Financing Administration (HCFA) within its five main divisions. However, the American federal constitution, based as it is on the separation of powers, ensures that there will be regulatory institutions within the legislative and legal branches of government as well as within the executive. The US courts and Federal Trade Commission, for example, have been active regulators since the 1970s. The Congressional advisory committee, the Physician Payment Review Commission, has since its establishment in 1986 reviewed this important aspect of professional activity. In addition each of the 50 states has its own local regulatory institutions apart from the licensing boards: in effect its own department of health services (though again, the formal title varies from state to state).

In addition to the professional and governmental regulatory institutions, the USA has a third grouping of potential regulators – the private sector. Most US health care is provided privately, through employment-related insurance schemes. Both insurance companies and large employers have become increasingly concerned at the rapid escalation of costs. This has turned them from passive payers into potential regulators. They have, for example, positively encouraged the rise of the new industry of private Utilization Review corporations. Utilization Review (UR) is the assessment of medical care to establish its appropriateness and its effectiveness. UR corporations, the newest players in the activity of regulation, are commissioned to check the necessity for medical treatment – for surgery, in particular – in an attempt by insurers and employers to contain their costs by tackling the issue of unnecessary treatment being provided by physicians. The growth of these UR corporations, who commonly have to be consulted before non-emergency hospitalization occurs, suggest that in a health-care system which is predominantly one of private provision there is room for private regulation too.

REGULATORY INSTITUTIONS IN GERMANY

The regulation of the medical profession in the Federal Republic is best understood as the result of the workings of two key features: the special significance of 'public law' institutions in the organization of the profession; and the importance of the wider political structure in Germany, especially the federal organization of government and the part played by the constitution and the constitutional courts.

The first important feature – the key role of public law bodies – brings us directly to the organizational structure itself. Public law bodies are organizations empowered by government to carry out regulatory functions, and given legal powers to carry out their tasks. They are widespread in the regulation of trade and industry in the Federal Republic. In medicine, two sorts of public law institutions are central. The first are doctors' 'chambers' or Ärtzekammern. The most important chambers are organized at the level of the individual Länder of the Federal Republic. The significance of the chambers is twofold: membership of a chamber is obligatory for any

practising doctor in the Federal Republic; and these compulsory organizations are the responsible bodies for key aspects of the regulation of professional life.

The chambers reflect a particular German philosophy of self-regulation.
They are governed by their membership, but have power over that membership which is backed by law, and they carry out functions delegated to them
by the governments of the individual states (Länder) in the Republic. The
most important of these functions is licensing which, nominally the duty
of the responsible Minister in the state government, is in practice done by
the physicians' chambers. From the powers to license doctors – in other
words to admit them to the profession – follow a number of other functions
related to the internal government of the profession. The chambers are the
relevant organizations for the control of medical ethics, the organization of
disciplinary tribunals and the continuing education of doctors.

The physicians' chambers may be considered the most important institutions in the organization of the medical profession, but they stand alongside
another key category of public law body, the Associations of Insurance
Doctors. The Associations owe their importance, as we saw in our historical
sketch, to reforms originally introduced some 60 years ago. They are at the
centre of the most important feature of the German health-care system – its
reliance on contributory insurance funds as a way of helping to cover the
cost of treatment for patients. The associations are organized regionally;
before re-unification between 'West' Germany and the German Democratic
Republic there were 18 in all. Unlike the case of physicians' chambers,
membership is not compulsory. However, in order to treat patients whose
care is covered by funds, it is necessary to be admitted to membership
and, since the overwhelming majority of the population is covered by
insurance, for most doctors in local practice, membership is in reality a
necessity.

It will be plain that the Associations of Insurance Doctors retain the
central position that they originally acquired at the start of the 1930s and
which we described in Chapter 3: in other words, their public law status
reflects their importance in standing between the doctors in local practice
and the insurance funds who are the ultimate source of doctors' incomes.
The Associations remain critical to the preservation of the independence and
power of doctors in local practice in the Federal Republic. As we will see
in Chapter 5 the conditions under which they carry out their functions is
the key to the continued maintenance of this power.

To Anglo-Saxon eyes the physicians' chambers are fairly recognizable
institutions: though they take a particular German form they carry out duties
not unlike those carried out in the UK, for instance, by the General Medical
Council and the various Royal Colleges. But the Associations of Insurance
Doctors have no immediately recognizable counterpart in either the UK or

the USA. In negotiating with the insurance funds over the pay of doctors, for instance, they are carrying out a function which in the UK is performed by 'trade union'-like bodies.

This does not mean, however, that pressure groups organized along the lines of Anglo-Saxon associations are unimportant. On the contrary, the division in the medical profession introduced by the separation between hospital and ambulatory care means that two separate associations representing different groups of doctors play an important role: a specialized association representing doctors in local practice (*Verband der niedergelassene Ärtze*); and an association representing doctors working in hospitals, the Marburger Bund. The latter is particularly significant, for two reasons. The first is that it does indeed perform the sort of 'trade union' functions carried out by doctors' associations in the UK, because doctors in hospitals, unlike their colleagues in local practice, are salaried employees. Second, the changing structure of the medical profession is making the Marburger Bund more important. In Germany there exists a long-term trend towards the employment of doctors in hospitals rather than in 'solo' practice in the community.

This description of the institutional structure of the medical profession in Germany conveys at first glance the impression of a highly fragmented occupation divided into a large number of separate organizations. In practice physicians are a good deal more institutionally cohesive than first appearances might suggest. The most important source of this cohesion is that many of the key organizations tend to share the same activists and leaders, so that the 'community' of doctors' leaders is comparatively small. In addition, there is a striking tendency for these leaders and activists to be drawn disproportionately from one, high-status part of the profession, the doctors in local practice. They dominate the professional regulatory organization and this in turn helps maintain the prestige of the solo practitioners.

The system is also held together by an institutional device introduced in 1977, a body usually known as the system of Concerted Action on Health Care. 'Concerted Action' is a body numbering about 70 representatives of the various interested parties to health care, including doctors. It tries to agree rates of increase of spending for the coming year. Though its decisions are recommendations, not law, it is important in integrating the doctors' organizations into the wider network of health-care policy institutions.

The organization of the regulation of the medical profession in the Federal Republic might be summarized as self-regulation within a statutory framework. It is this statutory framework which accounts for the second major feature shaping the organization of physicians – the role of the wider governmental and legal structure. The Federal Republic is both formally and substantively a federal system: in other words, the legal constitutional framework shares authority between the central government in Bonn and the separate governments of individual Länder; and this formal arrangement mirrors a society where these Länder exercise great practical influence over social and economic affairs. The Federal Republic is also a state founded on a constitution, the Basic Law. This Basic Law operates in a society where lawyers have high status, where most prominent public servants are trained in legal reasoning and where, as a result, legal rules play an important part.

All these features feed through to the organization of medical regulation. The most important doctors' organizations, the public law chambers and the associations of insurance doctors, are based, we have seen, on the Länder or on smaller regions. In the cases of both the chambers and the associations there exists German wide federations of the separate institutions, but in both cases the most important processes take place within the individual organizations at Länder or regional level. In other words, the decentralized, federal structure of the German political system is reflected in the decentralized, federal structure of the system for regulating doctors.

This is reinforced by the prevailing legal framework. In the case of the Chambers, for instance, it is the Land government which is the relevant regulatory authority. Indeed, in general the government in Bonn has few significant executive functions in the field of health care. It is, however, important as the shaper of the overall regulatory structure, and this structure is marked by a high degree of legal elaboration. This is an inevitable consequence of a system which assigns the regulation of medical care to bodies, like the Chambers, membership of which is compulsory and the structure of which is governed by law. But it is also a reflection of more general aspects of the legal system in the federal Republic – notably of the importance of the Basic Law in the attribution of rights and duties, and of the constitutional courts, both at the level of the whole Republic and of the individual Länder, in interpreting the meaning of the Law.

In summary, the distinctive features of the structure of regulation in the Federal Republic are as follows: the central role played by public law bodies, who act under legal powers delegated from government; the importance of law and statute in shaping the way organizations work; and the geographically decentralized structure of regulation, reflecting both the formal organization of the federal political system in Germany and, more generally, the actual extent to which authority is decentralized away from the federal capital in Bonn.

CONCLUSION

Our purpose in this chapter has been to provide a basic outline of the institutions of regulation in three countries, a preliminary to a discussion of the substance and impact of regulatory processes. From these sketches, three points should be noticed. The first of these recalls a feature which is now emerging as one of the most important characteristics of this comparative exercise: the national political structure within which the regulation of the medical profession takes place deeply influences how regulation inside the medical profession is organized. The most striking instance of this is provided by the contrast between the unitary structure in the UK, and the federal organization of regulation in Germany. Second, these structural differences are reinforced by a related factor, the different roles played by the constitutional traditions in affecting the organization of regulation. The mere possession of a written constitution is not itself crucial: we see that in both the USA and the UK, privately organized pressure groups, the AMA and the BMA, are central to regulation. But Germany again emerges as special, with the central role played by public law organizations in the regulatory structure.

Perhaps the single most important feature to be noticed in these sketches, however, is similar to that observed at the end of Chapter 3. Just as there is no single historical route by which the regulation of doctors has developed, so there is no single national institutional pattern. Every country has to organize so as to carry out the regulatory tasks identified in Chapter 2; but each country organizes differently. This organizational diversity should make us wary of blanket generalizations about the power of doctors. Of course, diversity in organization does not necessarily mean that other aspects of regulation will not show common patterns. It may be that in respect of both processes and outcomes the regulation of the medical profession in these three countries is indeed characterized by similarity rather than differences. This is something we will examine in Chapters 5 and 6.

FURTHER READING

The main UK regulatory institutions are the General Medical Council, the British Medical Association, and the various NHS authorities headed by the Department of Health. The GMC produces a very useful Annual Report on its activities and its organization is outlined in Stacey (1989). Baggott (1989) contrasts its very small number of 'lay' members with the situation on other UK bodies which regulate professional activities. The GMC and BMA are criticized as having excessive regulatory powers in chapter 4 of Gould (1985). Ham (1992) has good chapters (4–6) on the policy processes of both the Department of Health and the sub-national Health Authorities.

Raffel and Raffel (1989) provide useful and fairly detailed material on all the major US regulatory bodies, including the internal organization of the federal Department of Health and Human Services. Campion (1984) is the official history since 1940 of the American Medical Association, and so needs to be read with some caution when interpreting events. Pages 1–80, however, cover the essential basics of the AMA's organizational structure. State licensing boards are examined in Cohen (1980), and in Gross (1984). The rapid growth of Utilization Review machinery has led to a call for it, too, to be regulated – see Field and Gray (1989).

On German regulatory institutions in English, see Moran (1990) for an overview. Heidenheimer (1973), though dated, brings out the distinctiveness of the 'public law' nature of the doctors' organizations in a comparison with the USA. Döhler (1991), though analytically more advanced than a student would expect to read, has the virtue of being both up-to-date and of comparing the UK, USA and Germany. Part of Döhler (1989) provides a brief, simple sketch of the main organizations. Katzenstein (1987) is the best source on the wider national political system which shapes German institutions. Karcher (1990) describes some of the problems consequent on re-unification. 'Concerted Action' is outlined by Henke (1986).

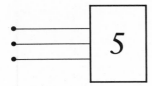

THE PROCESS OF
REGULATION

INTRODUCTION

From the previous chapters we now have an overview of several key aspects
of the regulation of doctors: we know from Chapter 1 the outlines of the
three health-care systems where our doctors work; in Chapter 2 we discussed
the chief general issues in regulation, and how these are linked to particular
questions about the regulation of doctors; from Chapter 3 we discovered
how the regulatory systems in the three countries have evolved historically;
and in Chapter 4 we sketched the main institutions concerned with regulation. But all this leaves a large gap in our understanding of the regulation
of doctors: we as yet know little of the *process* of regulation. This chapter
therefore describes how regulation actually works in the three countries that
are our concern; and it concludes by drawing out the common patterns, and
the differences, brought to light by comparison.

   The phrase 'the process of regulation' actually refers to two features:
the content of rules and how they are made. We could hardly understand
regulation if we knew nothing about its content. Fortunately, we already
have a framework for examining and comparing regulatory content, provided by the four regulatory 'tasks' identified in Chapter 2: regulation of
entry, of competitive practices, of market structures and of pay. Describing
how these tasks are tackled in three different health-care systems allows us
to compare key aspects of the regulatory process. But understanding

regulation involves more than understanding *what* rules are made; it also involves understanding *how* they are made and put into effect. In this latter connection we will want to bear in mind the concerns raised in Chapter 2 – notably, how far regulation differs radically between countries or how far, alternatively, the regulation of doctors forms similar patterns regardless of country. Many points of comparison are of course possible, but one especially significant feature was described in Chapter 2: it concerns the relative importance of the state in regulation. To recapitulate, we distinguished between three models: independent self-regulation where the state plays little or no part; state-licensed self-regulation, where the state licenses groups like doctors' associations to carry out the tasks of regulation; and state-directed regulation, where government agencies do the job directly without intermediaries. One of the questions we will want to ask of the four 'tasks' in our three countries is, therefore, which of these three 'models' best describes the way regulation is carried out?

GERMANY: A FRAGMENTED SYSTEM

It is sensible to begin our discussion of how the four regulatory tasks are carried out in Germany at the beginning of a doctor's career – the point of entry into medicine. Any aspirant doctor has to surmount two main hurdles: the barrier to qualification; and then the barrier actually to practising as a physician.

Regulation of entry

The most striking feature of the way entry into the study of medicine is regulated in Germany is its decentralized nature. Medical courses are run in higher education institutions, and these institutions are controlled by the individual Länder. There exists a *numerus clausus* – a mechanism restricting the numbers who can enter the medical faculties – but this has not prevented a huge growth in the numbers of medical students: in 1950 there were 12 400 students on medical courses; by the mid-1980s the figure exceeded 84 000. This flood into the study of medicine is due to three factors. First, the perceived rewards of medicine have been very high, thus attracting applicants. Second, in German universities there is a long tradition of relatively open entry: historically, students who matriculated – fulfilled the formal entry requirements – were entitled to attend. (The rise in numbers studying medicine is only part of a bigger growth in numbers in German universities: in the previous Federal Republic total student numbers rose tenfold from just over 128 000 in 1950 to some 1.34 million 35 years later.) This has meant that, while the *numerus clausus* exists, there are powerful sources of resistance to really stringent limits. Indeed, the *numerus clausus* is more a belated response to the flood of medical students than an effective way of containing their numbers. Third, the fact that decisions about restricting entry to medical courses are taken by the separate Länder who control education policy in their own territory means that it has proved exceptionally difficult to adopt any nationwide restrictive policy.

In Germany, as in most other countries, successfully completing a course of study is only the first stage in entry to the medical profession. After formal qualification all German doctors spend a period in hospital practice. Until recently, for the majority this was a prelude to the most important and desirable part of a medical career – working in local practice. Employment in a hospital is the first point of entry to the professional career, and still a precondition of eventually setting up in local practice. The ability of medical graduates to progress through this point of entry is a function of a number of features: the extent to which provision is made for 'probationary' places; and the extent to which hospitals demand the services of doctors. In both cases in recent years the demand for places has greatly exceeded the supply: estimates of the present levels of unemployment among German doctors range as high as 15 000. In other words it is at this stage, rather than at the stage of entry to study medicine, that the main barriers to entry to medical practice exist.

But the really significant career move for a doctor lies in the next stage after hospital work – entry into local practice. To understand why this is so we need to describe the status and function of local practitioners in Germany. The doctor working in the 'main street surgery' is a far more significant figure than the traditional GP in the UK. Indeed the local practitioner is the kingpin of German medicine. In the Federal Republic most local practitioners are not 'general practitioners' – they are specialists in particular branches of medicine, and well paid specialists at that. Entry to this lucrative and prestigious sector is the preferred destination of most German doctors. Formally, entry is lightly regulated. The real key to being able to set up in local practice is not the act of finding a surgery and putting up a brass plate on the door; it is being accepted into the membership of the Association of Insurance Doctors which exists in each Land (state) of the Federal Republic. Although a tiny minority of doctors practise outside the Associations, for the overwhelming number membership is an absolute precondition of being able to function as local practitioners. This is because the Associations organize payment for treating those patients who are members of insurance funds. As we saw in Chapter 1, the cost of health care for nearly every German is covered by a fund; entry into local practice and entry into the appropriate Association of Insurance Doctors is therefore virtually one and the same.

Since membership is a key to a lucrative career there have, not surprisingly, been efforts to regulate entry. The insurance doctors' law of 1957 fixed the maximum numbers of doctors at a ratio of 1 per 1500 population. This was challenged in the Constitutional Court by an association which represents the interests of hospital doctors, who naturally saw a threat to their members' right to progress into local practice. The Court, which interprets and enforces the 'Basic Law' (the Federal Constitution) struck down the restrictive provision in 1960, on the grounds that it violated constitutional provisions guaranteeing citizens the right freely to practise their professional vocation. That judgement in effect established what is, by UK standards, a very free system of entry. The consequences were twofold: increases in the numbers of doctors working in local practice; and, since doctors naturally gravitate towards the most affluent and pleasant areas, a striking geographical imbalance in the distribution of medical care. The judgement thus bequeathed to Germany the twin problems of oversupply of doctors nationally, and their undersupply in poor districts – like deprived city areas – where medical care is most needed. A prolonged debate throughout the 1970s and 1980s culminated in a law activated in 1987 which for the first time introduced planning restrictions over the geographical distribution of doctors admitted to the insurance doctors' associations. The limits are nevertheless comparatively slight: at the geographical level of whole Länder (which commonly embrace both rich and poor areas) the Insurance Doctors' Associations can restrict entry, but only to limited groups of doctors for limited periods, and only to half of all planning areas.

The regulations governing entry to the medical profession in the Federal Republic are thus relatively liberal. There is nothing like the system we will find in the UK, where there are tight central controls over entry to medical courses and close regulation of the geographical distribution of local general practitioners. At the point of entry the German medical profession is truly a 'liberal' profession. Despite this formal ease of entry into local practice, however, the sheer numbers of medical graduates produced by the universities has meant that there is a considerable blockage in the hospitals. The numbers working in hospitals now, for the first time, outnumber those in local practice; and hospital work, from being only a staging post on the way to a career in local practice, has for increasing numbers of doctors become their long-term career destination.

Regulation of competitive conditions

There is an obvious link between the regulation of entry and the regulation of competitive conditions, if only because a restrictive policy on entry is one of the most effective ways of controlling competition in any market. But there are two other aspects to the regulation of these competitive conditions: that concerning the relations between doctors and other providers of health care; and that concerning relations between members of the profession itself. We examine each in turn.

It is worth remembering that protecting doctors against competition from other providers of health care is a key factor in regulation. There is no 'natural' divide between the services provided by a doctor and those provided by others; on the contrary, the history of the establishment of medicine as an organized profession involved creating precisely those barriers against other health-care providers. These barriers remain contested in Germany. Much to the annoyance of doctors, for instance, pharmacists market many routine medical services, such as testing for blood-pressure levels. The profession has developed two key sources of protection against external competition. The first is the 'Chamber' organization described in Chapter 4. Membership of chambers is compulsory for anyone practising as a physician in Germany, and membership is open only to those who fulfil prescribed criteria – notably completion of the standard courses of academic and practical physician training.

The second barrier to competition is provided by the control doctors exercise over finance. Recall that almost every German covers the cost of medical treatment through a health insurance fund. We will see in a moment – under the 'regulation of pay' below – that doctors' organizations exercise tight control over the payment of their own members who work in local practice. In effect virtually every service provided by a doctor is paid for by the funds, and members of funds have direct access to the services provided by doctors. For other groups providing health care the position is very different. No other group of providers can directly bill the insurance funds for their services. This means that providers who are not physicians can only directly acquire custom from patients prepared to pay out of their own pocket – an insignificant proportion – or from patients referred to them by doctors. In effect, doctors are the 'gatekeepers' regulating access between patient and other health-care providers. The only exception to this is midwives.

Within the profession itself an important distinction must be drawn between conditions in local practice and those in hospitals. We have already seen that the barriers to entry into local practice, though they have been raised a little in recent years, remain relatively insignificant. There is nothing like the aggressive US advertising for custom, but patients have a great deal of choice: there is no requirement, as in the UK, to register with a particular practitioner; there are numerous specialists in local practice; and patients are in practice free to approach almost any doctor for a consultation.

This freedom of choice extends, however, only to treatment as an out-patient – 'ambulatory care', as it is called in the jargon, to distinguish it from the 'stationary' care provided for in-patients of hospitals. Here there exists one striking restriction on competition. It consists of the so-called monopoly of ambulatory treatment which is enjoyed by doctors in local practice. This monopoly, which is enforced by law, for the most part forbids hospitals from treating patients except as in-patients. Even more important, access to hospital services for patients is usually only obtainable through referral from a doctor in local practice. Although a small number of doctors have the right both to engage in local practice and to treat patients in hospitals, in general there is a clear separation in the German system between 'ambulatory' and 'stationary' care.

This separation is perhaps the single most important regulatory barrier to competition in the German system. It helps explain why the local practitioners have been the most prestigious and – until recently – numerous group in the profession. It also helps explain one of the most unusual features of the German system to UK eyes: the fact that only a minority of those who work in local practice are 'GPs' in the UK sense. The typical local practitioner is a specialist, and the typical local surgery is a world away from the 'low tech' world of the British GP, who works with few more technically sophisticated instruments than a stethoscope. The separation of ambulatory and stationary treatment means that doctors in local practice in Germany occupy an immensely important position, both because they control access to hospital care and because they actually deliver much of the care which in the UK is done in hospitals. But the separation is not only to the doctors' advantage. It also increases the range of choice available to individual patients. They not only have direct access to specialist care by, so to speak, just walking off the street into the surgery; they are also not tied to a particular local practitioner.

Regulation of market structures

It will already be plain that in Germany the regulation of competitive practices is connected to the regulation of market structures. 'Market structures' refers to the way those who provide goods or services in a market can organize themselves for the purposes of provision – for instance, whether the rules permit or prohibit particular kinds of business enterprise, like limited companies. In the Federal Republic the rules are indeed highly restrictive. This is particularly true of the ambulatory sector. As we saw in Chapter 3 one of the central struggles in the history of German medicine concerned the effort to distinguish the profession of medicine from 'trade' and this has left an indelible mark on the way doctors organize their business. In the ambulatory sector the 'solo practitioner' – as the Americans would put it – remains dominant. Doctors are effectively small entrepreneurs. The 'corporatization' of medicine – as the employment of doctors by firms is sometimes called – is effectively prohibited in the ambulatory sector in Germany. Indeed not only is the organization of the market by firms prohibited, for a long time it was also very difficult even to form partnerships, so deeply embedded was the notion that the doctor should work as an independent professional. This prohibition has now been relaxed, but the dominant structure in the ambulatory care sector is still the doctor practising as a lone professional. However, the enforced separation of ambulatory from hospital care in the Federal Republic has in turn influenced the organization of these solo practices. Because a majority of solo doctors are specialists of various kinds, offering what by UK standards are sophisticated forms of treatment in the surgery itself, they need high levels of investment in technology. The 'solo doctor' is far from being a lone worker. He or she, even when not in a partnership, will head a team of employees, including paramedical professionals who will conduct many of the specialist tests on patients. Indeed a common complaint by payers in the German system is that 'overtreatment' of patients is encouraged because solo doctors have to support the elaborate support teams in their employ.

The solo doctor in Germany, then, is a small entrepreneur, but an entrepreneur who typically is an employer, usually of other health professionals. In the hospital sector the position is much more varied. Doctors are for the most part salaried employees, but their employers are as varied as the structure of the hospital sector. The hospital sector is divided into three more or less equally important sectors: publicly owned hospitals, chiefly run by Länder or by local communities; hospitals run by charitable organizations, like churches; and privately run hospitals, some of which are owned by doctors.

Regulation of pay

Pay determination has been perhaps the single most disputed regulatory issue in the German system. Nor is this surprising: modern health-care systems are labour intensive, and the biggest costs are labour costs. Regulatory systems are not neutral in their effects: some methods of deciding pay are more expensive than others. Hence systems of pay regulation are everywhere inherently controversial.

In the German case a clear division exists between the regulation of pay in the ambulatory and in the stationary sectors. In the case of the former, two features are central: the way doctors calculate the charges they make; and the way payments are made. In the Federal Republic the calculation of charges is done according to what is usually called the 'fee-for-service' principle. Every item of treatment which a doctor gives has a price attached to it. In order to fix the price there is a catalogue, applicable nationwide, assigning points to all the services given by the doctor – covering everything from a home visit to a complex surgical intervention. In separate negotiations between the Associations of Insurance Doctors and the Insurance Funds a monetary value is then negotiated for the points, giving a price for each service. The negotiations take place between these organizations because individual patients hardly ever pay doctors directly for treatment. Almost every patient seen by a doctor will present a certificate from the particular insurance fund of which he or she is a member. This is then used by the doctor as the basis of the bill for treatment administered.

Here we come to a key feature of the German system. The individual doctor submits no claim to the insurers; payment is made by the Association of Insurance Doctors. This is why, in order to treat patients who are members of insurance funds, membership of the Association of Insurance Doctors which is organized in each Land (state) is vital. These Associations not only negotiate how the 'points' are converted into money; they also negotiate a global sum which they receive from the funds. This they then use to pay their members, who submit bills based on the treatments they have given to patients.

It will be obvious that the Associations of Insurance Doctors are the linchpin of pay regulation in the ambulatory sector, because they negotiate the monetary values to be given to the points system, because they negotiate the global sum for care, and because they disburse that sum. In addition, the fact that they are the paymasters of their doctor members means that they have acquired a further important function: they are responsible for monitoring the claims made by doctors under these arrangements to ensure that no fraudulent or otherwise unjustified claims are made. Before the Health Reform Law of 1988 (operational from 1989) this control function was exercised fairly passively; it involved scrutinizing the returns of a tiny sample of doctors to discover how far their claims deviated from the average. Under the new law, however, the control function of the Associations was strengthened and widened: the proportions of doctors to be examined was raised sharply (to 2 per cent each quarter) and the range of treatments to be scrutinized was extended.

Beyond the ambulatory sector, in the hospitals, doctors are mainly salaried and pay is the result of collective bargaining. The fee-for-service principle applies, not in directly determining the income of hospital doctors, but in determining the income of their employers, the hospitals, because reimbursement from the Insurance Funds for the treatment of patients is according to that principle.

The regulation of payment in the German system has raised the major issue of cost containment. Although the level of spending on health care in the Federal Republic is not out of line with international trends given the wealth of the country, the pay of doctors, especially of doctors in local practice, is exceptionally high by international standards – indeed on most measures is outstripped only by the income of US physicians. In the minds of many – especially in the minds of the main payers, the Insurance Funds – this is connected to the 'fee-for-service' system. According to this argument paying doctors for each separate service they perform offers a powerful incentive to physicians to 'overtreat' patients, since income is directly determined by the volume of treatment given. If the argument is correct, there is of course also an incentive to perform the more lucrative treatments which are awarded high point scores, and to neglect the less lucrative services. The perception that the fee-for-service system boosts doctors' incomes is one reason why the control functions of the Associations of Insurance Doctors have been strengthened under the 1988 legislation.

USA – PLURALIST REGULATION

We have seen in Chapter 1 that US health-care provision is primarily a private-sector activity.

Regulation of entry

The AMA was founded in 1847 primarily to improve medical education. It set up a Committee on Medical Education at the inaugural meeting, and thus has a long history of involvement in the regulation of medical schools. In Chapter 3 its role in reducing the number of medical schools during the early part of this century was noted. Later it unsuccessfully opposed the involvement of government in the direct funding of medical education, a change which led to the number of medical school places doubling between 1965 and 1980 (and the number of physicians doubling between 1960 and 1983). Despite its self-regulatory activities aimed at controlling supply, the USA is now close to having a surplus of doctors as a result of this expansion of medical education.

Accreditation as a doctor is a prolonged process. By contrast with the UK and Germany there is no undergraduate entry into medical study. Medical schools are for those who already have a college qualification. Acceptance to enter medical school remains fairly competitive. Despite the recent expansion, there has continued to be about twice as many applicants as there are places. In addition, the medical schools cannot guarantee that their products will be able to practise as licensed doctors, for each of the 50 states has its own licensing board, established by law. In general, however, state boards have traditionally been dominated by the profession – so much so that there have been instances of boards simply handing over their responsibilities to the local medical society, the local branch of the AMA. On the other hand, the inability of the Association to obtain a monopoly for allopathic medicine (the treatment of disease with drugs having the opposite effects to the symptoms – nowadays called 'orthodox' medicine) means that medical lists usually include qualified osteopaths and sometimes chiropractors.

The lack of any national standards for medical education was partly rectified with the establishment in 1915 of a National Board of Medical Examiners (NBME). This drive against the low standard local commercial medical schools which littered the USA, was inspired by the AMA and funded by the Carnegie Foundation. Many state boards accepted NBME standards, then later all accepted a Federation of State Medical Boards examination which used NBME questions and gradings of candidates but left to local decision issues such as the frequency with which the examination could be taken. In addition, there still remain inter-state variations in the requirements for residency training in hospitals, and for periodic re-accreditation of doctors: for example, 21 states require proof of some further training before re-licensing, a requirement opposed by the AMA. For US medical graduates, then, market entry is governed by a mixture of conditions – national examinations coupled with local variations in their interpretation and in the detailed criteria for licensure.

The shortage of doctors in the 1950s and 1960s led to a large-scale use of foreign medical graduates, not always properly screened. When, after legislation in 1976, a new examination was established, there was an 80 per cent failure rate. This tightening-up of requirements, largely a response to the doubling in size of domestic medical schools, was a move made by government with the AMA acting in positive partnership. The ostensible reason was uncertainty about foreign medical schools' standards but in practice the AMA was naturally keen to exercise more control over the supply of doctors. The drastic cut-back in the acceptance of foreign medical graduates affected many American-born doctors as well as those with other nationalities, because large numbers who failed to get into US medical schools had emigrated to train, usually in nearby countries such as Mexico or Puerto Rico.

Differences between state licensing boards also extend to the disciplining of doctors: in 1987 Kansas took action only against one doctor in every 2 000 whereas the more vigilant West Virginia took action against one in every 120. Sometimes state law helps explain such extreme variations of disciplinary activity. California, for example, has a Board of Medical Quality Assurance which operates with its hands tied behind its back. It can review only a specific complaint against a doctor, but to revoke a licence it needs to show 'a pattern of gross negligence' and is unlikely to be able to do so unless there are many specific complaints lodged against the same doctor, a fairly unlikely scenario.

Finally, few state boards have checked the record of the doctor in other states before granting a licence to practise, and there has been a lack of coordinating machinery to prevent a doctor moving to another state after having his or her licence revoked or suspended. This has been a significant gap in the institutional machinery. It should soon be closed following 1986 federal government legislation to establish a National Practitioner Data Bank of information about all disciplinary actions taken by hospitals, insurance companies, or state boards. In this instance a clear failure of self-regulation has been overcome by government-led and directed regulation.

A fairly definite pattern of the regulation of market entry and exit has now emerged. There is a strong tradition of self-regulation in which the AMA plays a prominent part. This covers the accreditation of medical schools, organization of examinations, and dominance of many state boards. But self-regulation has not always worked, and where the failure has been very marked there has been state involvement – the public funding of medical education as a stimulus to its expansion, and the Practitioner Data Bank to make state-hopping more difficult being two prominent instances.

Regulation of competitive conditions

Most US doctors are in solo practice, self-employed, and earning a high income through a system of fee-for-service payments. The profession has always supported this system, and has sought to strengthen it through a regulatory process which has deliberately limited competition between physicians, has discouraged the acceptance of alternative treatments such as those of chiropractors, and has opposed salaried doctors, systems of provision based on capitation rather than fee-for-service, and utilization review procedures which question a doctor's autonomy of diagnosis and treatment. In every case the extent of self-regulation has been reduced in the last 25 years – by government, by private-sector payers, or by both acting in partnership.

Professional rules of behaviour for many decades banned advertising. This ban has now successfully been challenged by the same governmental bodies that have increasingly become involved in several aspects of professional activity which had always been left to the profession itself to regulate. Governments began to argue that existing rules about competitive practices were contrary to the public interest. The American Federal Trade Commission (FTC) used Anti-Trust Laws to charge the AMA and two Connecticut medical societies with unlawful restrictions on advertising, and in 1982 won its case in the Supreme Court. The AMA's formal published rules then had to be amended. So did some of its other rules about price-fixing, educational accreditation, and boycotts of chiropractors, following FTC activity over those issues.

Concern about steep and regular rises in health-care costs have led to the emergence of two new sets of institutions which regulate, or constrain, the freedom of doctors to practise: prepayment organizations and utilization review systems.

The growth of prepayment, in particular of Health Maintenance Organizations, has been quite rapid in recent years. In 1985 just under 8 per cent of Americans were enrolled in an HMO; three years later this had risen to 13 per cent. HMOs are the direct antithesis of the traditional fee-for-service approach to health care. Instead they are based on the concept of 'capitation' under which the organization provides all necessary care in return for a fixed annual fee. Often they employ salaried doctors, though the more recent variation, known as Preferred Provider Organizations, pay a list of approved doctors a set discounted fee. Their attraction is their record of cost containment, and the vast majority of large employers offer at least one choice of HMO as part of their benefit package, usually at a premium level of about 25–35 per cent below that of fee-for-service rates.

HMOs and other systems of what is often called 'managed care' are not, of course, regulatory institutions *per se*. But their impact on the competitive conditions within which doctors operate is becoming increasingly apparent as they grow. They represent a challenge to the traditional medical cultures of doctor-determined fees and of treatment plans which pay no regard to costs. They are thus having the impact of a regulatory body, albeit still at the margins.

So, too, are Utilization Review (UR) programmes, again as a response to the cost explosion. UR focuses on the appropriateness of care, and is increasingly being used by insurers and businesses as well as by federal and state Medicare and Medicaid bureaux. Hospitals have developed large in-house systems and there are private specialist corporations who offer services to businesses. The methodology is an examination of medical notes to check whether or not a treatment plan proposed by a doctor is appropriate.

Utilization Review has been found to cut hospital expenditure by 11.9 per cent and total medical expenditures by 8.3 per cent, and research has shown that the specialist companies save almost $9 for every $1 they charge. As with 'managed care', UR programmes thus represent a challenge to the traditional freedom of doctors to treat and to charge as they see fit, acting independently and subject to no check or medical audit. These government and market-led developments are regulating the practice style, behaviour and salaries of US doctors. Their impact can be seen not just in terms of percentages but in the fact that they are unpopular within the profession because of the challenge they represent to the traditional concept of medical autonomy. Until their arrival US doctors had practised in an unchallenged setting with minimal accountability to peers for the standards of care provided, and with a need merely to satisfy the patient who is for the most part not in a position to judge due to ignorance of modern medicine and medical autonomy.

Regulation of market structures

Regulatory control of market structures is extremely limited in the USA. Doctors can practise wherever they want and in what groups or partnerships they choose, subject only to some pressures from within the profession. For example, the AMA has a long history of opposing corporate medicine, or salaried employment within a factory or workplace, and this has helped deter the spread of that type of health care.

Even the small-scale inducement of newly qualified doctors to work in shortage areas has now ended. From 1972–90 a system of scholarships to medical students was linked to a duty to serve for up to four years in a very rural under-doctored location. This small-scale programme was always informal and scarcely regulatory, and was wound up by a simple announcement from within the Reagan administration.

As we have seen, the medical market structure centres on the office-based solo practitioner. This was central to the ideology of the US profession and remains the dominant influence in medical politics. Many office-based physicians are specialists, and they work simultaneously in hospitals by virtue of 'admitting rights'. Any one specialist may well have admitting rights to several hospitals, and the hospitals generally only employ on a salaried basis physician assistants or junior doctors.

This pattern of domination by the solo practitioner is gradually being challenged by a number of developments encouraging the spread of salaried doctors. The steady rise of HMOs was charted above and seen as a response to the cost explosion, partly fuelled by the traditional ability of solo practitioners to determine their own fee-for-service, a market structure seen as offering an incentive to maximize treatment. Another response was a rapid growth of Physician Assistants. From 1980 to 1985 their numbers rose by 40 per cent, and they are attractive to hospitals seeking cost reductions, as well as to solo practitioners expanding their practices.

If recent trends continue, the dominance of the solo practitioner will soon be challenged. Excluding federal doctors working in the Veterans or Indian services, by 1985 some 26 per cent of physicians in the USA were employees, and no less than 47 per cent of younger (under 45 years of age) doctors fell into that category. In addition, increasing numbers of 'fee-for-service' physicians are partly abandoning their right to determine the size of fee by contracting with collective payers (such as Preferred Provider Organizations or some large companies) to provide a given level of health care for a fixed payment. The traditional market structure is clearly under pressure.

One solo practitioner in eight has simultaneously had ownership interests in health-care facilities (such as hospitals, clinics and laboratories) to which they refer patients. This poses ethical problems of conflict of interest. The only regulations, AMA rules, have done no more than suggest that doctors who own facilities to which they might refer patients should inform the patient of this financial interest when asking them to agree to be referred – a modest guideline which appears to be of little effect. An official investigation of Medicare patients in 1989 found that referrals and services were provided at a 45 per cent higher level when the doctor had a financial interest in a health-care facility. In its report the Office of Inspector-General – a federal government agency – made six proposals for change, including stronger utilization review arrangements and even the prohibition of certain types of referral, but the matter was left to the AMA to regulate. The Association's response was a lukewarm restatement of its existing regulatory guide-lines, coupled only with a vague general call for disciplinary action where unethical referral practices took place.

Market structures, then, are changing in the USA. The changes reflect wider developments in the provision of health care – the search for cost containment in particular – rather than attempts by regulatory institutions to positively alter the market structure. Formal regulations remain as scarce as ever, but the profession continues to organize itself and to espouse policies on the basis of the dominance of solo practice, the centrality of fee-for-service, and the system of admitting rights to hospitals.

Regulation of pay

The regulation of pay in the USA has recently proved perhaps the single most contentious issue in the whole area of medical regulation. American doctors are the highest paid in the world and are among the most prestigious professionals in US society. The US health-care system is also the world's most expensive and is often accused of failing to deliver value for money in terms of acceptable indicators of patient care. And it is as frequently alleged that one of the chief reasons for this is the method of paying doctors.

American doctors historically set their own fee levels. There were no regulations and a free market existed. Their opposition to the introduction of Medicare and Medicaid was so strong that the federal government in 1965 in effect accepted unregulated fees by a political agreement enabling physicians to continue to bill the federal and state authorities, charging what were their 'usual, customary and prevailing' fee levels. Insurance companies, too, have accepted this tradition of doctor-determined bills.

As costs rose, both within the public programmes and in the (larger) private sector, doctors began to have to negotiate with the major institutional payers. Until the 1990s the outcomes of struggles about physician fees continued to favour the profession in that the institutions (federal and state governments, insurers and employers) did not challenge the fundamental right of the profession to determine its own fee levels. Instead of regulating doctors through the imposition of fee schedules they accepted cost-shifting systems (deductibles and co-payments) involving patients sharing the burden directly. Indeed, many patients found it necessary to take out back-up insurance policies to cover such eventualities and by 1990 it was estimated that the average senior citizen was spending as large a proportion of his income directly on health care (by paying for treatment or by taking out a 'Medigap' policy) as before 1965, despite 'benefiting' from the Medicare programme.

About 40 per cent of all spending on health care in the USA comes from the public purse, and governments in the 1980s led the attack on the non-regulation of physician payment. This culminated in federal legislation in 1989 to introduce fee schedules for Medicare payments from 1992.

Fee schedules as such were not new – many states had used them for a decade or more for Medicaid payments. But what was new was the imposition of fee schedules based not on the claims of doctors under the 'usual, customary and prevailing' agreement, but on a fully researched analysis of the relative value of different treatments. A ten-year study of 7000 medical procedures had sought to measure four major dimensions of physician input: time; mental effort and judgement; technical skills and physical effort; psychological stress. Known as RBRVS (Resource-Based Relative-Value Scales) the results came as a bombshell. Most types of surgeons were adjudged to be extremely overpaid whereas diagnostic interviews and family practice were heavily underrewarded.

The new Medicare fee schedules will thus regulate part of doctors' pay in a revolutionary way, and legislation includes a number of safeguards which add to the amount of regulation. The profession benefits from the incorporation of a 'budget-neutral' model guaranteeing no change in total physician fees. The regulators, in return, plan to prevent having to pay for an increased volume of activity. If surgeons, for example, find more hernias to repair or babies to deliver through Caesarean section, fees will be adjusted downwards and 'overpayment' clawed back.

This degree of formality and abandonment of doctors' rights to set their own fee levels is a major development in USA health care in that it moves the focus of regulatory emphasis from hospital costs (at centre-stage throughout most of the 1980s) to physician costs.

Though Medicare accounts for only 17 per cent of US health spending, these formal regulations about doctors' pay are very significant in that they could lead to the widespread insistence on fee schedules by insurance companies and business. It is thus conceivable that a key historical feature of the so-called private market approach to health care in the USA might be 'regulated away' in the 1990s.

UK: PREDOMINANTLY CENTRALIZED

Britain has a long tradition of strong unitary government and centralized regulatory and policy-making institutions. Though elected local authorities are responsible for the detailed provision of several parts of what is known as the 'welfare state' (education, social services, for example), the regulation of doctors, and the organization of the NHS, comes under the auspices of appointed bodies such as the General Medical Council and the NHS Management Executive. Additionally, as we saw in Chapter 4, the profession organizes itself through the national Medical Association and Royal Colleges. This centralized set of institutional arrangements impacts upon all four regulatory tasks.

Regulation of entry

The first really effective barrier to practising as a doctor occurs at the point of entry to UK medical schools. Competition to enter from school leavers is intense, and high educational qualifications are needed: indeed, few university degrees require higher ones. This intense competition reflects the regulatory control over numbers of entrants which is exercised by the Department of Health. On the basis of advice from a Medical Manpower Standing Advisory Committee – which the Department appoints – the Secretary of State for Health prescribes the total annual intake to medical training.

Decisions on both the number of medical schools and their size are influenced by medical opinion as well as by financial considerations (medical schools are extremely expensive and UK students are not expected to contribute to the basic costs of training). The profession has been broadly content to see admissions, and hence the supply of UK-trained doctors, fairly tightly restricted. Indeed, one of the most striking features of doctor supply in the UK is the very narrow bottleneck established by the control over entry to medical school. The UK has relied heavily on foreign medical graduates, both in hospitals and in local practice, and the regulated expansion of medical schools has maintained that reliance. From time to time reports into the shortage of doctors have resulted in more medical school places being made available.

The medical profession controls the choice of entrants to medical schools and the contents and methods of instruction. Admissions officers who process applications are medical academics. The basic syllabi are invariably designed to ensure the approval of the General Medical Council, whose education committee plays an important part in curriculum design. Graduates are thus certain of acceptance onto the GMC's statutory medical register.

The licensing by the GMC of foreign medical graduates is rather more problematic. The Council operates by, in effect, maintaining a list of 'recognized' foreign medical schools, and itself amends that list from time to time (for example, graduates of the University of Malaya medical school in Kuala Lumpur have not been acceptable for registration since 1989 after extensive review, over a number of years, of the arrangements for teaching and assessment). In addition the Council sets a stiff clinical and a language examination.

The GMC is bound by quite detailed Parliamentary statutes. Foreign medical graduates, for example, are by law given either 'limited' or 'full' registration – the latter being on a par with fully registered UK graduates. Though the GMC has been left to itself to determine how a doctor moves from limited to full recognition, it has not been given the power to merge the two systems. The introduction of a single form of registration for all overseas doctors, favoured in principle by the GMC, would require a change in the law and so could only happen with the explicit approval of Parliament. Other examples of this quite detailed involvement of UK politicians with medical regulation will arise later. As in this case, the distinction between procedural rules and policy content is crucial – there are formal, legal rules about types of registration but the quite formal though more flexible (in not needing the approval of a higher authority) rules about the criteria for registration are left to the regulatory institution itself to design and promulgate.

The GMC is also responsible for medical discipline and it determines what is and is not acceptable professional conduct. Its disciplinary procedures are governed by statutory rules to a very detailed degree. For example, complaints first go through a screening process before being heard by the relevant GMC committee, and lay GMC members cannot be involved in that process by law – so the enlarged lay membership of recent years is circumscribed in its activities. Similarly, the legal rules prevent the GMC from investigating patients' complaints about the attitudes of doctors or about their general standards, because disciplinary matters have to involve an incident of 'serious professional misconduct'. Though the Council has made moves to widen its interpretation of this key phrase so as to include serious cases of rudeness, only about one complaint in eight received by it goes forward for investigation by the GMC's disciplinary committees. Some, at least, of the other seven might well be considered by the local appointed health authorities – which provide the NHS – if the complainants approach them following advice from the GMC, but health authority disciplinary powers are limited and only the GMC can remove a doctor from the medical register.

A strong element of central control exists in the later stages of market entry as well as at the outset. The most desirable medical posts have been as hospital consultants, usually obtained only after a long apprenticeship in more junior hospital grades. The crucial influences shaping a doctor's chances of obtaining a consultant post are not just those of existing consultants and academic doctors, who play a prominent part on the local appointments committees, but also those of central government which determines the exact number of consultancies in each specialty and each region.

This picture of the profession with little apparent independent control over market entry, though with considerable control over discipline and market exit, is not the whole story. Government decisions on the funding and size of medical schools, and on the numbers of consultants in different specialisms, are heavily influenced by medical opinion. Government employs medical advisers as civil servants, and operates a network of formal advisory committees which give the profession consultative status over a wide range of issues. Perhaps even more important is that, for rather different reasons, government and the profession broadly agree with regulatory policies which restrict domestic market entry and make UK doctors a scarce and hence a valuable commodity.

Regulation of competitive conditions

The picture of an amicable partnership between government and the profession has traditionally also applied to much of the regulation of competitive conditions in UK medicine. The referral system and separation of hospital from ambulatory care is a notable illustration of this partnership. As we saw in Chapter 3, the profession itself reached a self-regulated agreement more than a century ago about the distinction between hospital and general practice doctors. Competition between the two types of doctor was avoided by hospital doctors restricting their activities to hospitals and general practitioners referring patients when there was a need for more specialized advice and treatment than could be provided in the community. When the government introduced the National Insurance Scheme in 1911, and then the National Health Service in 1948, it found it convenient to adopt, rather than challenge, this self-regulated division of labour. The profession was strongly opposed to both the 1911 and the 1948 reforms, so it made political sense for the Government to seek as much common ground as possible. The division and referral system seemed to work, and the Government was not searching for more competition but for better access to care. Later, the 1989–91 NHS reforms also accepted the hospital-general practitioner distinction. Even though these latest reforms sought to introduce more competition and market forces, this was restricted to competition within each medical grouping, not between them. Almost certainly one key reason for not trying to restructure the whole profession in 1989–91 was because the Government was convinced that the referral system was cost effective, economic, even cheap to operate.

Until the late 1980s the profession had very successfully minimized competition between hospital specialists and between GPs. Indeed, the Government had rarely made any comment about the existence of non-competitive regulatory practices such as professional bans on advertising, and at GP level, government regulations were based on the need for patients to register with one doctor by not making it easy to change GPs. At hospital level, the system of payment by fixed annual salary did not offer any incentive to seek extra patients, and so prevented competition between specialists for trade. The 1989–91 reforms, and other contemporary moves by the Government, changed the picture somewhat. At the hospital level, the new regulations separated the provider (the hospital) from the payer (the local health board or authority). The aim was to make hospitals compete with each other to offer the 'best' service, with cost being a key factor as health boards had fixed amounts to spend on buying care. The pressure was thus on hospital doctors to become more cost-effective or to be more productive. Their clinical autonomy over diagnosis and treatment was not directly challenged, but they were, in effect, being regulated to produce more for their salary.

Regulation was much more direct at GP level. New rules imposed by the Government after discussion with (but not with the total agreement of) the profession made it a good deal easier for patients to change GPs, and this was widely publicized. In addition GPs were made to produce leaflets and annual reports, and the new contract they had with the NHS imposed many other requirements on them which had previously been matters left to their discretion (compulsory regular check-ups for the elderly, for example). Simultaneously the ban on advertising by GPs, hitherto a piece of self-regulation, was overturned.

Nudged by the Government, the Monopolies and Mergers Commission – a government agency with a brief to encourage competition in the economy – produced a report in 1989 on medical advertising which was, perhaps surprisingly, welcomed by both the Government and the profession. The government welcomed it because it recommended that GPs be allowed to advertise; the profession welcomed it because it endorsed the principle that self-regulation should continue and that specialists be still barred from advertising (because this would undermine the NHS referral system). In 1990 the General Medical Council altered its rules and introduced an informal set of guidelines which it described as 'a loose set of rules and principles' to be reviewed and firmed up after a year's experience of GP advertising. Indeed, the chairman of the GMC Standards of Professional Conduct committee stated that 'there are no rules; there are general principles saying claims have to be legal, decent, honest and truthful'. Shortly afterwards the BMA produced its own code, which was also flexible. Neither self-regulatory body – GMC nor BMA – favoured advertising, but Government pressure could not be resisted.

The example of advertising is more widely applicable to the degree of formality of regulations about competitive practices. In general in the UK, these regulations are formal in that they are published, but fairly informal in that they are reasonably easily and frequently changed because they are ratified by the regulatory institution itself rather than after a process of obtaining the external agreement of other, higher bodies. In May 1990, for example, the General Medical Council at one single meeting was able to amend the regulations on advertising by doctors; on direct access to specialists (making this even harder for patients to obtain); and on advertising by private healthcare providers. This last change was totally unrelated to the Monopolies and Mergers Commission's report and was designed to prevent private healthcare providers from making invidious comparisons with one another and with the NHS.

Regulation of market structures

A critical part of the 1946–8 negotiations between the Government and the profession related to the ability of all doctors to undertake private work alongside their NHS commitments, and of GPs to retain their status as self-employed professionals operating through a contract with the NHS. In both cases the Government acceded to professional pressure and produced a regulatory framework which has the appearance of being state-led but is in practice as much the creation of the profession.

Political bargaining has therefore led to a situation in the UK where doctors ostensibly employed 'full-time' by the NHS can also undertake private work. In addition, the NHS employs a large number of doctors on a part-time basis. Hence the vast majority of hospital consultants and of GPs have additional earnings from private work – consultations and operations at the specialist level; medical examinations for insurance companies and even for other government departments at the GP level. Often these activities can be undertaken in NHS premises under the negotiated agreement of 1948.

The self-employed GPs have increasingly grouped together in partnerships in order to share the expense of overheads such as receptionists, nursing staff, and office costs, though there still remains a sizeable minority of solo practitioners. The popularity of partnerships, usually of between two and six doctors, has led to the production of formal regulations about succession: the rest of the partnership has (as one would expect, given the self-employed status of GPs) the right to select their own new partner when one dies, retires or leaves. When a single-handed GP leaves, however, the local health board chooses the successor.

The geographical market structure of general practice is strictly regulated by the national Medical Practices Committee (MPC). Though self-employed, GPs cannot just 'put up a plate' anywhere and undertake NHS-paid work. (Notice the contrast with, for instance, the much freer German system.) The MPC issues strict criteria, based on the average list size of the local GPs. Areas are classified as 'restricted', 'intermediate', 'open' or 'designated' and applicants are treated according to the classification of their area of choice – they are prevented from practising in a restricted area, for example, but offered financial incentives at the other end of the scale, in a designated area. The result is a fairly equitable distribution of GPs, and a closely regulated market structure which ensures that list sizes vary only between around 1500 and 2500 patients (the average GP has slightly under 2000).

The regulation of pay

UK doctors have two broad sources of income: from the NHS and from private practice. The processes and extent of regulation of the two sources, not surprisingly, are very different.

The private practice income of most GPs is derived from undertaking non-NHS medical examinations, vaccinations and reports. Most GPs follow a fee schedule determined by the BMA's private practice and professional fees committee. The schedule is merely 'recommended' and here is a classic example of professional self-regulation with no powers of sanction on those who choose to determine their own fees, though payers which are institutions (the Department of Social Security, for example, uses GPs to undertake medical examinations as part of the test of eligibility for certain benefits) will expect GPs to use the set fee schedules, and will only pay those amounts. Individual payers, on the other hand (such as the would-be tourist needing inoculations) lack knowledge of the BMA fees, and have no bargaining clout.

Junior hospital doctors have few opportunities for private practice. But at least two-thirds of the UK's 17 000 consultants have significant incomes from private work – an average £38 000 in 1991, or almost as much as their *basic* salary from the NHS (but see below for merit award income). This average conceals wide variations, with the leading 20 per cent doing most of the work and averaging no less than £95 000 from private work. Here there are no clear fee schedules, and any regulatory activity is predominantly by the insurance companies, which are increasingly seeking to keep costs down as average claims ran well ahead of inflation in the 1980s. But these insurers have yet to go beyond exhortation. Clear clinical protocols and fee schedules remain no more than a vision of the future, though the steady rise in private health insurance, and the poor financial results of some insurance companies make such moves towards market-based regulation increasingly likely to happen.

Almost all GPs and junior hospital doctors, and around half the hospitals' consultants, rely heavily on income from the NHS. The regulatory process is essentially one of bargaining between the government and the British Medical Association, supplemented since the early 1960s by an independent adjudicatory panel – the Review Body on Doctors' and Dentists' Remuneration (known as the DDRB). The Secretary of State for Health negotiates with the medical profession about the structure of the payment system and the Review Body gives a monetary interpretation to the agreed payment system in normal years. Occasionally the structure of the payment system is not agreed but imposed by government, as happened in 1990 when the basis of GP incomes was altered by the imposition of a new contract. The BMA opposed the increase in capitation payments per patient and the introduction of target payments for vaccinations and cervical cytology tests (a GP had to reach a set of targets to obtain any fees for this work). It preferred the previous approach of a higher basic allowance and of a fixed fee per inoculation or smear test, regardless of the numbers of patients involved. However, it was overruled. Nevertheless, since 1948 agreement on the pay structure has been the norm, with disputes restricted to the amount of income increases rather than their distribution.

The DDRB, the pay review body, was established when the two sides – doctors (the BMA) and government – were unable to maintain their post-1948 relationship which was based on compromise and, albeit sometimes reluctant, agreement about both the amount of increases and the distribution of doctors' incomes. The DDRB in effect arbitrates, taking evidence from both the BMA and government, and reporting annually. As part of the agreement behind its establishment, government by convention accepts the report – ministerial pledges on this were an important consideration when the profession indicated a willingness to accept the new machinery. Occasionally full implementation is either delayed or phased in on the grounds of incompatibility with the immediate economic situation, but no government has yet sought to reject a Review Body report: indeed, the system has subsequently been introduced for other public-sector professions, notably for the pay of nurses.

These NHS pay processes are based on collective agreement. The individual GP, junior hospital doctor or consultant has very little freedom to determine his or her NHS income. The two latter groups are on fixed salary scales applicable universally; the GP receives fixed amounts though these can be increased by taking on more patients or undertaking more activities which are paid for on an 'item of service' basis. However, there is a national notional 'pool' for GP pay, and if all GPs did increase their activities so that the pool ran dry in any year, the following year's pool would be reduced by the amount of 'overspend', and the excess payments would be 'clawed back' from every GP by an overall adjustment of fees. This happened quite markedly in 1991–2. The 'pool' for 1990–1 was heavily overspent as GPs sought to enhance their incomes under the imposed new contract, in particular by obtaining fees from running new health promotion clinics and from doing more of their own night visits rather than calling out a commercial deputizing service. (UK GPs have a duty at all times to provide necessary care to patients. Many had chosen to use commercial deputies at night. From 1990 they received three times the fees for attending in person, a deliberate inducement to which many reacted positively.)

For hospital consultants – or some of them – the collective agreement and set salary is supplemented not only by private practice earnings but also by a system of individual rewards or bonuses within the NHS. Another aspect of the 1948 agreement was the establishment of Distinction Awards, or additional payments to consultants with 'outstanding professional ability'. A highly confidential system of 'peer review' was established, and four levels of Award developed. By 1990 some 35 per cent of NHS consultants were in receipt of an Award, and by retirement some 60 per cent were holding one. Most Awards enhanced the basic salary of around £40 000 by about 18 per cent, but some added as much as 95 per cent. The traditionally profession-dominated Advisory Committees have since 1990 had several health authority general managers added to their membership, but the register of Award holders is available only to consultants. The names of Award holders remain entirely confidential, even though Awards are met from within the general public spending allocation for health.

CONCLUSIONS

In the UK the centralized political system, the national organization of the medical profession and the existence of an NHS have all helped shape the process of regulation. There is a mixture of self-and state-regulation, with the latter largely restricted to pay and to issues affecting the structure and operation of the NHS, which has a duty to ensure free access to necessary health care. The profession is left to police entry and exit, and most regulatory issues are determined by negotiated agreement between government and the profession.

'Variety' is the watchword of this chapter: variety in the regulation between countries, and variety within any one country, between the four regulatory tasks examined. That variety extends to two main areas, which we now examine in turn: the nature of the regulatory process, and the influences shaping that process. On the first of these we shall look especially at how far 'rules' are formal or informal, and at which of the models identified earlier in the book best makes sense of that process: self-regulation by the profession; state-led regulation; or government regulation.

On the question of what influences shape the regulatory process, we look at four 'candidates': the structure of government; the wider economic system within which regulation is provided; the 'regulatory culture' of each country; and the health-care system itself.

Types of regulation

Formal and informal regulation

The degree of formality of the process of regulation offers us one way of comparing the regulation of doctors across different countries.

Regulation can be formal or informal. By formal we mean based on established, published rules. These rules may be found in laws, approved by and only changeable by the legislature (in the UK, by Parliament; in the USA, by Congress or the state; in Germany, by the two houses of the legislature, the Bundestag and Bundesrat). This is the most formal of all regulation. Or the rules may be drawn up and approved by the regulatory institution which makes it quite clear that all its decisions on particular cases will be based on its rules. Less formally, there can be codes of conduct, guidelines or recommendations which indicate the general thinking of the institution but do not bind it or the regulated. Finally, decisions can be entirely informal, based neither on written rules or guidelines nor on any precedents created by previous decisions.

Because regulation directly affects the ability of doctors to practise and to earn a living, it is unlikely to be operated in an entirely informal manner. This would be unacceptable to the profession. In addition, most of the key regulatory institutions identified in the previous chapter are large-scale organizations. This almost inevitably means that, if rules have not been imposed upon them, they will generate bureaucratic methods of operating and will be inclined to produce their own written rules. How they interpret their rules is a matter for later in the book. Here we are concerned more with the extent to which they are responsible for writing their own rules, and with the specificity of those rules as this gives an indication of the ability of regulators to act flexibly.

Regulation is not equally formal across all the four areas on which this study focuses. For example, the formality and specificity of regulations about market entry and exit (i.e. disciplinary activity) are in all countries very marked. The accreditation of medical schools in the UK and the examination system used by state boards in the USA is a known, detailed regulatory arrangement. On the other hand, what amount to regulatory processes about market structures are much less formal. Indeed, as we saw particularly in Germany and the USA, they are sometimes by-products of the systems of payment for health care and as such are nowhere codified. Even the referral system in the UK is not easy to identify in a formal set of rules – rather, it was inherited and utilized by the NHS, not created as part of it.

The formality of pay arrangements also varies. In the USA – at least until the new Medicare fee schedules take root – there is an extraordinary degree of informality behind the apparently highly bureaucratic method of billing for every activity. The UK contrast in terms of NHS pay is almost total – a Review Body, published written evidence and very detailed recommendations which, by convention, are accepted by government.

The message is quite clear. Although there are some important national differences, it is dangerous to make sweeping statements about the formality or informality of national regulatory processes, beyond a few broad generalizations such as the greater involvement of government in Germany and the UK in the regulation of doctors. Much better is to examine particular tasks of regulation on the basis that there is unlikely in any one country to be a pattern of a formal–informal balance applicable to each task. In brief, our evidence does not support the hypothesis, sketched in Chapter 2, that there are distinct national styles of regulation.

Self-regulation or state regulation
At first sight there are only two types of regulatory institutions: those established by government to oversee certain aspects of doctors' activities, and those created by the profession itself. Hence the distinction made between state-led and self-regulation in the title above and in some of the literature on professionalism.

By now we know that such a simple, neat categorization of regulatory institutions makes little sense. Certainly those who are involved in regulation do not see things in this way. A new member of the UK General Medical Council said this (in its Annual Report for 1989) after a year in office: 'Self regulation is a privilege afforded to few groups in our society. I believe that the nature of medical practice necessitates the existence of a strong independent regulatory body.' This apparent confusion between self-regulation and independent regulation is understandable. On the one hand, the GMC was established by government as a public institution. On the other hand, the GMC has always been dominated by doctors, with little more than a token lay membership.

	Government-led	Profession-led
Source	GMC	
Composition		GMC
Rules	GMC	

Figure 5.1 State- and self-regulation continuum: the GMC case.

This example of the British GMC, which could apply equally to the US state boards, suggests a need to refine our categorization of regulatory institutions. At one end of a continuum there may well be institutions which are entirely governmental in terms of their establishment, their procedures and policies (or rules) and their membership. At the other end are the totally professional bodies, usually medical associations or their offshoots. In between are mongrel institutions – some set up by government but dominated by doctors to varying degrees; some with the appearance of being self-regulatory but involving governmental nominees or representatives. In the case of the GMC in the UK this distinction between source, composition and rules places it at three different points on the continuum, as Figure 5.1 illustrates. Set up by government, its members are predominantly doctors, and its rules are a mixture of statutory requirements and GMC designed codes of conduct and rules of market entry (as we saw earlier in the chapter).

It is possible to analyse every regulatory institution in a similar manner, and place it at different points on the continuum. But for our purposes the important point is to assess the broad extent to self-regulation in each country, and to indicate the need to look beyond the façade of any regulatory institution before drawing conclusions about its true nature.

At first sight, UK regulatory institutions are state-led. The General Medical Council, the Medical Practices Committee and the NHS pay negotiating machinery and local health boards all stem from governmental decisions. Regulatory processes, therefore, appear to be both centralized and political.

In reality this description is misleading. The BMA plays a key role in all four regulatory tasks, sometimes through having representation on significant committees and at other times through the rules and guidelines it, itself, issues. It ensures that health-care decisions made by government are seen as 'political', and acts as in effect an institutionalized 'opposition', questioning the policies and proposals of government.

UK regulation of doctors is, then, by and large of the mongrel variety. The façade of state-led institutions gives way to an interior of marked doctor influence, and the earlier remark made by a new GMC member becomes understandable – the GMC is an apparently 'independent' statutory body, but to all intents and purposes its dynamics are predominantly those of professional self-regulation.

US regulation is in some ways quite different because many of the institutions start by being placed at the other end of the continuum, as purely self-regulating. The AMA and its offshoot joint committees with other professional groups dominate many aspects of medicine in a way which the BMA does not. The presence, noted earlier, of a single federal representative on the 23-member Accreditation Council for Graduate Medical Education is merely token (and not just because the federal representative has no vote). Furthermore, the medical capture of many state licensing boards means that they are only government-led in terms of their creation.

But self-regulation is on the defensive in the USA. As the author of the official history of the AMA has put it: most doctors 'ardently' want 'a basically private medical care system' with patients and doctors 'free to choose' and with minimal governmental activity (Campion, 1984, p. 506). Hence the Association fought the public funding of medical schools and the introduction of Medicare and Medicaid programmes for the poor and elderly – and lost. Later the key issue switched to cost containment, and again the AMA's wishes to retain the traditional system of doctor payments have not been successful, with new Medicare fee schedules having received legislative approval. On these issues, at any rate, the traditional notions of overwhelming doctor power have had to be re-thought. Likewise, professional control of supply ended with the federal funding of medical schools to encourage expansion.

State-led regulation has also been prominent in the area of competitive practices, with the successful activities of the Federal Trade Commission and courts in ending professional boycotts and cartels. And the USA has also witnessed a further type of regulation – by the market. The rise of 'managed care' (HMOs, for example) has begun to impact upon market structures as institutional payers have sought to contain their costs by searching for better value for money than that offered by the traditional system of professional self-regulation.

In Germany, too, the traditional extent of self-regulation has begun to be questioned. There the key issue has been the non-accountability of self-regulation. The payment system is dominated by the Insurance Funds and the Associations of Insurance Doctors. Both sets of associations are legal creations, subject to the final oversight of the state. Both are also in principle subject to the internal control of their members. In practice, they tend to be run by small élites. The funds, for example, are dominated by their full-time officials. Although there is a formal apparatus of democracy, with provision for the election of governing bodies by the mass of subscribing members, participation is low and the influence of the ordinary member minimal. The positions the Insurance Funds take up in negotiations with the doctors over payment are largely determined by their officers – though of course these officers in turn may be motivated by the desire to defend patients' interests, as well as by the fear that members will protest if subscriptions rise too sharply. As far as government is concerned there is a substantial deficit in control – a deficit which institutions like the 'Concerted Action' (see p. 63) can hardly be said to have made up. The most important and visible part of the health-care budget – the bill which the Insurance Funds have to pay for care, and therefore the contribution levels which their members have to make – is set by a process of bargaining over which patients, and the patients' elected representatives in government, have little control. This, of course, contrasts sharply with governmental control of supply through the open-access policy which operates in higher education, and which has led to a surplus of doctors.

The search for better regulation has resulted in a marked degree in Germany of 'licensed self-regulation' through a wide range of non-governmental public law bodies. We saw that membership of the doctors' 'Chamber' at Land level, and obedience to their discipline, is a condition of being able to practise medicine. We have also seen that while membership of the Associations of Insurance Doctors is not formally obligatory, in reality few doctors in local practice could survive without joining. And we have seen that, especially in the vital matter of pay regulation, the Associations and the Insurance Funds are the most important institutions in determining what happens. It might be asked how a system so decentralized manages to function at all – and indeed, one of the main problems in the German system: is its apparent inability to produce radical reforms. The forces of fragmentation, however, are partly nullified by the two other features of the system domination by doctors and the existence of a highly cohesive network of regulators. Although many institutions share the regulatory tasks, doctors are the most important actors. If we had to sum up the German system in a single phrase it would be 'licensed self-regulation by doctors' – and by doctors enjoying a large measure of discretion under the terms of the licence. Now we turn to what influences the process of professional regulation in medicine.

Influences on regulation

The structure of government
This refers both to the wider structure of the national political system and to government of the health-care system in each of the three nations. Much of the regulatory process is an outcome of how a nation allocates the

regulatory function between different parts, and different levels, of the state machine. Perhaps the most obvious example of this in the preceding discussion is provided by the case of market entry. It is plain, for instance, that the essential clue to the character of market entry regulation in Germany lies in the federal system: in the way the control over medical education is in the hands of the individual Länder, through their control of university education. In contrast, in the UK there is central control of medical education, both of finances and student numbers. In the USA the highly fragmented organization of medical schools has involved central (federal) government acting as a facilitator for expansion through the injection of public funds since the 1960s.

In Germany the supremacy of the Basic law, or constitution, has also been a fundamental influence on the way entry to local practice is controlled. We saw that attempts to regulate numbers of local practitioners were destroyed by the decisions of the Constitutional Court in 1960, which ruled such regulations to be a violation of the safeguards on occupational freedom in the Basic law. In contrast, the UK has had a long history of centralized manpower control, with government and the profession acting as partners happy to keep the supply of doctors down. US federal involvement, by contrast again, has been designed to reduce the stranglehold on supply which had been wielded very successfully by the profession.

The wider economic system

A second obvious major influence on the nature, processes and extent of medical regulation is the prevailing economic system within which doctors practise. The clearest example of this lies in the contrast in competitive conditions between our two European cases and the USA. The substance of regulation in the UK and Germany has limited the amount of competition within the profession and protected doctors from the competition of outsiders. Indeed, this impulse to protection can be said historically to have been the most important driving force behind the formation of the medical profession. In the US the effort to limit commercialism and competition was also present, but its long-term influence has been much weaker. The more competitive and commercialized character of US society has produced a more commercially-orientated system of professional organization. Doctors compete much more obviously for business; health care is much more consciously operated as an industry in which commercial rules of corporate rationality are to the fore.

The regulatory culture

The third important extraneous influence on regulatory processes is what is best called *the regulatory culture* itself. In this connection there are striking contrasts between all three of the countries used as cases in this study. Many observers have remarked on the distinctive regulatory culture of the USA. To quote Vogel (1986, p. 267):

> The uniqueness of the American approach to regulation is the one find-ing on which every cross-national study of regulation is in agreement. The American system of regulation is distinctive in the degree of oversight exercised by the judiciary and the national legislature; in the formality of its rule-making and enforcement process, in its reliance on prosecution, in the amount of information made available to the public, and in the extent of the opportunities for participation by non-industry constituencies.

Vogel is here writing largely about the regulation of large corporations, but it is plain that many of these characteristics are apparent in the regulatory process among doctors. Perhaps the most important instance of this is the control of market structures. Competition among doctors is, we have seen, in some ways remarkably fierce in the US system. But it is also plainly true that the regulation of market practices is both extraordinarily and unusually governed by processes of litigation. In other words, there is exactly that com-bination of minute rule enforcement and adversarial relations that Vogel has identified as characteristically American.

When we turn to the UK we observe a very different regulatory style, and this undoubtedly influences the way competition is controlled. The courts have been comparatively unimportant (though as we shall see in Chapter 7, this may be changing). Ethical standards and medical discipline are in the hands of a quasi-public body, the General Medical Council whose delibera-tions, though quasi-judicial, are controlled by the profession. Competitive conditions are closely controlled, but these controls have been relaxed by the most recent (1989–91) reforms – just as the Thatcher years saw a more general attack on the restrictive character of economic regulation in the country. Finally, in the German case we can see that the regulation of market structures reflects exactly that country's unique dual system of regulation – the combination of extensive juridification with extensive delegation to private institutions. Thus the law prescribes the institutional forms, and also specifies a range of restrictions like the separation of ambulatory and hospital work. But it also delegates to a series of public law bodies – notably the Länder-based Chambers of Doctors, and the Associations of Insurance Doctors – the power both to make the regulations and to enforce those regulations governing market standards.

The health-care system?
Finally, many observers might have expected a fourth 'influence' on regulation to have been emphasized: the organization of the health-care system itself. Our question mark reflects scepticism about this. In

Chapter 1 the very different systems of the NHS in the UK, national insurance in Germany, and market-based or pluralist health care in the USA were outlined to illustrate the setting within which doctors actually have to practise. However, we have subsequently discovered that in the UK many of the regulatory processes and institutions pre-date the NHS, and that centralized health care through governmental responsibility for its provision reflect the wider political move to a welfare state and the unitary nature of the UK constitution. Similarly, German fragmentation of health-care provision and medical regulation accords with the country's wider political processes, as does the endurance of the US market-based approach, and the reliance under the separation of powers on state governments to both regulate market entry and to pay for care for the poor. In general, then, we see the health-care system as a secondary influence, itself influenced by the structure of government, the economic system, and the general regulatory culture of a country.

We conclude by re-emphasizing one of the main themes of this book: while the regulation of the medical profession is undoubtedly in part shaped by the particular needs and demands of the profession itself, and by the needs and demands of health care, it is also the product of larger forces. The regulation of market entry, of market structures, of competitive practices and of pay reflect wider institutional structures and distinctive national regulatory cultures. This is not to say that medicine and doctors do not exhibit also some regulatory patterns which recur in different countries. These common patterns will be examined in Chapter 7. In the next chapter, however, we look at the outcomes and impact of regulation.

FURTHER READING

For Germany, many of the subjects covered in this chapter are not discussed in English-language sources. The discussion of entry regulation, in particular, relies on German-language material (see below). An exception is van den Busche (1990). Ham *et al.* (1990) provide a brief, up-to-date review of pay and cost issues. Hurst (1991) and Webber (1991) both focus on the same issues, with special reference to reform attempts. Schneider (1991) concentrates in particular on the cost and competitive structures of the German systems. Henke (1991) and Deutsche Bundesbank (1991) both analyse the payment system, in Henke's case discussing the potential problems created by unification. Iglehart (1991a, b) is especially good on pay, and on recent reforms.

In the large German literature, Lubecki (1987, 1989) is authoritative on entry to 'local practice'. Oldiges (1988) discusses the constitutional problems of regulating entry. Deppe (1987b) is the authoritative source on the history of entry regulation and its effects in the profession. Gockenjaan (1987) discusses the evolution and structure of competitive conditions. Mark (1986) is an overview of the competitive and institutional structure, focusing especially on pay arrangements. All the issues examined in this chapter (entry, competition, pay) are discussed in detail in Deppe (1987a) where a highly sophisticated neo-Marxist interpretation of the medical profession is developed. Breyer *et al.* (1987) are an especially valuable source on the hospital system. Webber (1989) relates all the regulatory issues to the attempt to reform the system at the end of the 1980s.

Challenges to the monopoly powers of US doctors, traditionally used by them to limit competition, have revolved around a series of court cases based on the anti-trust laws. These are charted and discussed by Havighurst *et al.* (1989, pp. 49–64). Folland (1985) finds no conclusive evidence on whether advertising of physicians' services enhances or impedes competition. The rise of 'managed care' largely through Health Maintenance Organizations is measured by Gold and Hodges (1989). The complex new system of Medicare fee schedules (based on Relative Value Scales) is outlined by Ginsburg *et al.* (1990), and compared to the German (and Canadian and French) payment systems by Rodwin (1989). The American Medical Association's most recent reviews of the licensing and accreditation processes are in *JAMA* (1988a, b). Wilsford (1991) examines the changing political strategies of US and French doctors in chapter 9, noting that in the USA politicians continue to seek to accommodate the views of physicians whereas in France they have been forced to take direct action. Stone (1977) compares the 1970s' attempts at peer review in the USA (the Professional Standards Review Organizations, or PSROs) with post-War 'Economic Monitoring' in (West) Germany and sees both systems as essentially self-regulation. Ermann (1988) is an excellent account of the rise and evolution of peer review systems in the USA over the last 40 years.

On entry into UK medical schools and the licensing of overseas doctors see the Annual Reports of the General Medical Council. The final chapter of Klein (1989) traces the background to the reforms of 1989–91, which included both the new GP contract and the introduction of an 'internal market'. The reforms themselves are reviewed by Day and Klein (1991) and Enthoven (1991). Strong and Robinson (1990) critically examine the 1980s' record of doctors as managers of services in part two. Ham *et al.* (1990) compare the 1989–91 UK reforms with developments in other countries, including Germany and the USA. Godt (1987) compares the strategies adopted to meet professional resistance to change through the 1980s by UK, German and French governments as they sought to contain rising costs. On doctors' pay and conditions of service, see chapter 4 of Harrison *et al.* (1990). The UK system of Distinction Awards is outlined and made less secretive in Department of Health (1990).

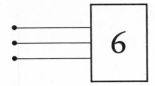

OUTCOMES OF REGULATION

INTRODUCTION

We now know that there are different styles and processes in regulating doctors. The history, the institutions, the influence of doctors and the content of regulation vary from country to country. Does this variety of systems matter? To the historian and the student of administrative behaviour it certainly does. Doctors and would-be doctors also need to be aware of the setting within which they will operate. But other observers have rather different interests, for their concern will be with the impact or outcomes of regulation. These outcomes might or might not vary from country to country. We saw in Chapter 2 that there are common issues of regulation such as accountability, standards, efficiency and effectiveness which apply everywhere. Such issues might be tackled in contrasting ways, but with similar results. Alternatively, the results – or outcomes – might also contrast.

This chapter builds on Chapters 3 to 5 by examining outcomes, or the consequences of regulation. It does this by focusing in turn on three main groups of actors in a modern health-care system – doctors, patients and those who pay for health care (in a different guise patients can also be payers, of course; but most payment is by organizations – governments, insurance companies, businesses). In the case of each actor in turn the single key question to be asked and answered is whether regulation is beneficial to them or whether it operates against their interests. An initial hypothesis about the impact of regulation on each of our four issues (pay; market entry; market structures; competitive practices) is examined by applying the empirical material presented in Chapters 3 to 5.

THE IMPACT OF REGULATION ON DOCTORS

Historically, doctors wanted regulation. In the UK, in particular, the advent of a medical register after the 1858 Act weeded out two-thirds of those claiming the status of doctor. In the USA, too, the later development of regulatory machinery was seen by doctors as a way of reducing competition from 'alternative' medicine. In Germany regulation was also seen as the key to reducing competition from other suppliers of medical care.

Our hypothesis is, then, that doctors benefit from regulation in a number of ways. Regulation of medical education and of the acceptability of qualifications can control the supply of doctors. Competition, both from other professions and from within the profession, can be limited. Regulatory machinery and processes can ensure that doctors control their own behaviour and discipline, and influence their own pay.

From the doctor's perspective, then, regulation can be a powerful support force. It need not be a limitation of professional autonomy – indeed it can enhance that autonomy. It can be used to give a profession both self-esteem and public status. Beneficial consequences can result from a positive public image which sees the profession as acting in the interests of patients. The most obvious benefit is that doctors receive delegated authority from government to regulate their own affairs. They work in partnership with the state, and themselves determine what are, and are not, acceptable practices.

This opening hypothesis sets up the Utopian world of regulation, as seen through the eyes of doctors. It establishes, in effect, the medical state – separate from the political state. Medical policy is seen as a matter for doctors to determine. Now let us look at how far reality and Utopia correspond.

Market entry

Contemporary regulation of doctors, which we now examine, almost inevitably does not match the hypothetical state. The ability of the profession to control supply, for example, reveals an extremely varied outcome. The relatively open access to German medical schools, and the restricted access to UK medical schools was noted in Chapter 5. The result is that Germany has, per thousand population, almost exactly twice as many practising physicians as the UK, and there is a significant surplus of doctors in Germany. A phenomenon virtually unknown in the UK – medical unemployment – has for some years been common in the Federal Republic.

UK and US doctors, indeed, were so successful at regulating the output of medical schools that both countries experienced acute shortages of doctors in the post-War period. In each case there has been a large-scale dependence on foreign medical graduates to fill the gap. Through the General Medical Council in the UK, and through state licensing boards and the AMA in the USA, some controls over entry have been imposed. In the UK, from the doctors' perspective, these have succeeded in preventing any over-supply which might seriously depress incomes and reduce career opportunities. In the USA the outcome is less clear. Government involvement in medical school funding from the early 1960s led to a dramatic expansion of schools and places and has now created, in many parts of the USA, a surplus of doctors. In this case the replacement of self-regulation by direct government involvement has quite dramatically altered the regulatory outcome within a fairly short time, and the profession has been unable to restore the balance of supply and demand by pruning medical school places or by stopping the entry of foreign graduates, though standards have been tightened.

Competitive practices

Regulations restricting open competition between doctors have been remarkably successful in the UK and Germany, in two quite separate ways. In each case the outcome has been quite different in the USA.

First, in the UK and Germany there has been no open advertising of services. This situation also applied throughout the USA until the Anti-Trust enforcement activity which followed the Goldfarb Supreme Court case of 1975 – the Goldfarb decision was that professions were not exempt from federal Anti-Trust Laws. Thus the courts and federal government agencies took over the regulation of competitive practices from the profession, and sought to extend competition. The outcome actually remains mixed in that in some localities doctors responded by agreeing amongst themselves not to advertise in the newspapers or telephone directories (for example such an agreement is operated by the St Louis Metropolitan Medical Society, which has about 2500 members).

In the UK, the Government has also intervened to increase competition by pressing the profession to accept advertising by GPs, as we saw in Chapter 4. Again, the outcome is patchy, partly because the new rules have only applied since 1990. Certainly there is as yet no perceptible rush by GPs to advertise in newspapers or telephone directories, though there is a trickle of activity such as leafleting an area, especially where a doctor re-locates premises or sets up a new practice.

The second aspect of competition and regulation relates to the boundaries of medicine. Historically all three countries drew tight boundaries through regulation. In the UK those boundaries remain sacrosanct, with doctors retaining their monopolistic rights to treat (under the NHS anyway – the truly private patients can go to whomsoever they wish) and to prescribe medication. Thus osteopaths, chiropodists, therapists and nurses work within the NHS under medical control, and homeopathy can be practised by a doctor only, and not by a homeopathic expert who lacks a medical training. Though ostensibly a triumph for self-regulation, this monopoly has actually been reinforced by state activity – the creation of the NHS formally legitimized these tight boundaries.

In both Germany and the USA medical monopolies have been challenged. In the German case pharmacists, for example, are potentially serious rivals. It is already usual for routine tests – such as blood pressure checks – to be carried out in the pharmacy, and pharmacists widely advertise the services they offer. This intrusion into the doctors' domain has been made greater by policies designed to cut the cost of health care. Under cost-containment measures introduced at the end of the 1980s, for instance, German pharmacists are empowered to alter doctors' prescriptions if they judge that the same therapeutic effect could be achieved with a drug cheaper than the one on the prescription form.

US doctors have had to accept osteopaths as equals in many states since the beginning of the century, and in recent years have been legally ordered to end boycotts of chiropractors. In 1987 the courts found that the AMA and its members participated in a conspiracy against chiropractors in violation of the nation's Anti-Trust Laws. The AMA was ordered to distribute to each member a two-page summary of a Permanent Injunction Order and it did so by publishing it (*JAMA*, 1988c).

Market structures

UK and German doctors have successfully regulated a referral system which determines market structure and also reduces competition. UK GPs and German doctors in local practice act as gatekeepers to high-cost hospital services. In Germany direct access to hospital care by the patient is all but impossible – and treatment of 'out-patients' by hospitals is similarly restricted. The so-called monopoly of ambulatory care enjoyed by doctors practising in the community prohibits hospitals from offering rival services. The fact that patients must present themselves to a local doctor also means that the doctor is the 'gatekeeper' to the hospital, regulating the amount of business that hospitals enjoy.

The rule separating out-care from hospital care is probably the single most important regulation governing the structure of the market in Germany. It helps explain, for instance, why local practice has been the most prestigious and best paid part of medicine. And it also helps explain a striking contrast with the UK: in this country local practitioners are overwhelmingly general practitioners; in Germany, it is possible to walk into the surgery of numerous specialists and to receive their treatments without admission to hospital. In the USA, by contrast, the hospital-locality distinction is blurred, with specialists having both local offices and admitting rights to several hospitals. Thus paediatricians and gynaecologists have to compete directly for patients, whereas under a referral system the competition is internalized within the profession and the respect of colleagues is central. In another way, however, it is the UK market structure which has experienced a unique outcome of regulation. In both the USA and Germany the self-employed solo practitioner has remained the central feature of medicine, even though in both countries the rise of the hospital has created an alternative pattern of salaried institutional staff. In the USA, indeed, the solo practitioner was able to use hospitals to further a practice by obtaining admitting rights and working with patients when they required institutional care, though the recent rise of corporate chains of hospitals has somewhat threatened this, because such chains often employ salaried doctors. In Germany local practice as a solo doctor remains the apex of the career structure, and the formation of group practices has been strongly discouraged by doctors' organizations.

In the UK, in contrast, two developments have undermined the status and the numbers of solo practitioners. First, hospital work has for long periods been fashionable and general practice has been regarded as second best. After the 1965 GPs' Charter, agreed with government, this situation changed, and general practice became a popular choice of 'speciality' in the 1970s and 1980s, but the imposition by the Government in 1990 of a new and allegedly more demanding contract on GPs could possibly lead to a decline in the popularity of general practice. Certainly the consultant hospital post remains a much sought-after target for most medical students.

Second, in UK general practice there have been changes of working styles. In particular, working together in groups has become the norm in most areas, both urban and rural. Anything from two to as many as nine or ten GPs operate as a collectivity, sharing overheads and lists of patients, and able to choose their own new partners on the death or retirement of a colleague or the expansion of the group's workload.

Pay

Doctors' remuneration varies considerably from country to country. Using national average pay of all employees as a base, we find that in 1986–7, UK doctors' incomes stood at a ratio of 2.4 times average pay; German doctors' were at 4.3 times and American doctors' at 5.4 times. One reason for the differences, and for the relative wealth of American doctors, is the regulatory system and its impact on salaries.

The USA has largely continued to treat doctors' pay as a matter not requiring regulation. Hence bills have been based on the 'usual, customary and prevailing' charges of the doctor, a phrase accepted by government in 1965 when it introduced Medicare and Medicaid. As costs rose rapidly, largely due to the increased uptake of health care by the newly eligible elderly, handicapped and poor, fee schedules of a sort came in – but always with the important proviso that if the Medicare fee schedule did not meet the normal physician's bill, the difference could be charged to the patient. Hence regulated fees did not affect total income – at least until the late 1980s when a few states sought to stop this cost shunting, and when new Medicare fee schedules to commence in 1992 were introduced by Congress as part of the 1989 Budget.

This non-regulation of pay contrasts sharply with the German and the UK experiences. The German system described in Chapter 5, has had three distinctive outcomes. First, it rewards large groups of doctors extremely well, whether measured by German pay levels generally or by international comparisons of doctors' pay. On the latter, German doctors usually emerge as second only to US physicians in the 'pay league'. These figures, however, are averages concealing wide variations, and it is these wide variations which are the second important outcome of the German system. There is an especially large – and probably widening – gap between the high pay of those in local practice and the low pay of younger salaried doctors working in hospitals. The third result of the payment system is more political than economic. The 'fee-for-service' system described in Chapter 5 is highly contentious. Payers – especially the insurance funds – believe that it offers incentives to doctors and hospitals to 'overtreat' patients in order to maximize income. Whether accurate or not, this is a widespread perception. The result is constant argument about the payment system, and attempts by the payers to tighten-up regulation so as to limit doctors' opportunities to exploit the system for profit.

In the UK the approach has been the reverse of fee-for-service, through salaries for hospital doctors and capitation (a fixed payment per head for each registered patient) as the dominant feature of GP income. Hence in the UK there has been no financial incentive to over-treat; in the USA every financial incentive; in Germany likewise, though with growing efforts to control exploitation. The regulatory outcomes in terms of doctors' pay appear to have been as might be expected – and this apparent confirmation of the significance of the system is further attested to by the Canadian experience. In Canada government moved from a US-type pluralistic system of health care, to a national insurance system which included fee schedules. In 1970 Canadian doctors' incomes were comparable to those in the USA at fivefold the national average wage; by 1987 the ratio had fallen to under fourfold, and there was a flow of migrant doctors into the USA.

Doctors: overview

That regulation can and does affect doctors is now apparent. The outcomes of regulation are variable. There is no uniform pattern. US doctors, for instance, have benefited from the lack of income regulation whereas UK doctors have suffered income restraints under a governmental independent Review Board, whose recommendations have not always been immediately implemented in full. UK and German doctors have also been subject to a strict referral system and limited competition – both the consequences of self-regulation and internal professional agreement.

As to supply, in Germany neither doctors nor any other interests have been able to get firm control over the flood of entrants. We described the difficulties in Chapter 5, and the outcome is reflected in the rising numbers of doctors, and in the bottlenecks forming in the traditional points of entry to medical practice, the hospitals. Americans, too, lost their direct influence over supply some 30 years ago with the intervention of federal government into the financing of medical schools. In this case it is the UK profession which, despite from 1939 losing to government its control of the numbers of entrants to medical schools, has in effect, by its success in persuading government to restrict student numbers, retained what it would view as a desirable outcome of a slight shortage of doctors, making those that qualify from UK medical schools a scarce 'commodity'. Senior UK hospital doctors – the consultants – have been equally successful in preserving their status (and with it the considerable perks of merit awards and of lucrative private practice). There have been government attempts to alter their numbers, and the ratio of senior to junior posts as a result, but little has happened despite at one point a clear government–BMA agreement to alter the balance by creating many more consultant posts.

This last example illustrates an important general point about the outcome of regulation: it may be unintended or unexpected. Some years ago, for instance, the government and the BMA agreed to expand the numbers of consultants. But the expansion never happened, partly because governments were reluctant to add to NHS spending levels but also because the existing consultants were anxious not to see their élite status watered down by a flood of new appointments. Similarly Anti-Trust cases have not everywhere resulted in doctors' advertising in the USA. The lesson is that regulation can be sometimes side-stepped by doctors, and that the study of the actual outcome of regulation is at least as important as an analysis of institutions and their rules.

THE IMPACT OF REGULATION ON PATIENTS

Doctors, then, have initiated, welcomed, accepted and (occasionally) side-stepped regulation. They have also resisted it in certain instances, notably when it has involved a major overhaul of health care, as in the cases of the introduction of the UK NHS in 1948 and its reform in 1989–91, and of the US Government's adoption of Medicare and Medicaid in 1965. These are, of course, relatively infrequent examples, but they illustrate the natural professional preference for self-regulation (whether or not it is state licensed) over government-led regulation.

If, by and large, physicians accept the need for and extent of regulation, how should patients view the regulation of their doctors? Our approach is to test a set of working hypotheses which view regulation as a support for patients, because regulation can guarantee quality of care and treatment. Only qualified medical practitioners will be able to set up as doctors, and they will then be subject to ethical codes and disciplinary procedures. Regulation can ensure quality-control systems and geographical location to enhance access to care. Finally, regulation can prevent over-charging and over-treatment.

As in the previous section, these working hypotheses are, of course, idealistic. They presume that regulation is patient-centred whereas we already know that many outcomes accord with the interests of doctors, and these are not necessarily compatible with those of patients. On the other hand, we have also been aware of the professional claim that doctors act first and foremost in the interests of patients, a claim which has historically legitimized the close relationship between doctors and the state, and which has been accepted by the state as justification for systems of self-regulation. So we can begin our investigation of the impact of regulation on patients by assuming that regulation should be beneficial: that quality assurance should result from the plethora of regulatory systems identified in previous chapters.

Market entry

The accreditation of medical schools and examination of foreign medical graduates prior to their being licensed to practise are instances of regulations which patients view positively. Indeed, in both the USA and the UK there have been occasions when public pressure has caused the examination of overseas doctors to be tightened up – more because of language and communication problems than because of concern with clinical skills. Many patients would claim that the outcome of the regulation of supply has been unsatisfactory in that the profession has helped create acute shortages, and that both the UK and the USA have had post-War histories of many academically well-qualified school leavers unable to obtain a place in a medical school, while simultaneously there has been such a shortage of doctors that health care has depended on immigrant labour, sometimes from overseas medical schools viewed widely as less than first rate. Germany has not had this experience because educational regulation has favoured more open access to medical courses.

Patients are also concerned with market exit. They rightly expect regulation to include disciplinary codes and procedures, to ensure that doctors act properly and ethically, in accordance with the Hippocratic Oath. Do the outcomes of regulation accord with these aspirations?

There are certainly regulatory systems in place, as was noted in Chapter 4. State licensing boards in the USA and the General Medical Council in the UK can and do reprimand some doctors and strike others off the approved list. In addition there are local complaints procedures in the NHS and as part of Medicare and Medicaid systems. However, outcomes are, at best, patchy. In the UK, doctors are rarely struck off, and those that are have usually behaved improperly towards patients (commonly through sexual relations) or have offended against anti-commercial regulations (for example, by buying organs from live donors for transplantation). Scarcely ever are doctors disciplined for clinical incompetence, which is much more likely to be of concern to most patients. In 1992 the GMC for the first time took steps towards introducing the regulation of the clinical competence of practising doctors, by publishing a consultation paper.

The German experience shows the difficulty of assessing the impact of regulation on patients. Responsibility for discipline lies with the doctors 'Chambers', but negligence cases can also be pursued in the courts. In the 1980s there was a rapid growth of litigation, and for many years there has existed an association for the protection of patients' interests. But there is debate over the significance of all this: whether it reflects an increase in the damage done by doctors to patients; or whether it reflects increasing awareness of their rights by patients.

The US experience is unique in one respect. In some states there are very active licensing boards and consequently high levels of disciplinary activity; in others, discipline is much less strict. Thus in 1987 West Virginia's board took action against 1 doctor in every 120, whereas Kansas disciplined 1 in only 2000. Again, as in the UK, 'strikingly few' of these cases involved 'medical incompetence or malpractice' (Schwartz and Mendelson, 1989). Further evidence that regulatory outcomes are unsatisfactory in the USA is that more doctors have their personal assurance terminated or actually resign than are disciplined. The key regulators of clinical competence, then, are not the official licensing boards but are doctors' insurers against malpractice claims, and the courts which hear those claims.

Competitive practices

Regulation was commonly initially designed to weed out what were colloquially called 'quacks'. Today many who are excluded from medical registers are styled as providers of 'alternative medicine'. In the UK they all remain excluded from the GMC's Medical Register and tight professional boundaries based on the primacy of allopathic medicine have been maintained. In Germany the boundary is a little less clear, especially between doctors and pharmacists. In the USA there is variation. Commonly osteopaths are listed by state licensing boards, but chiropractors are not, despite recent court decisions banning medical boycotts of them.

In all three states the existence of tightly defined medical registers has commonly been seen as advantageous to patients, but is becoming a matter of increasing debate. The alternative argument is that tight boundaries reduce competition and reduce access to health care. Providers of alternative medicine compete at a disadvantage if NHS or Medicare patients cannot use their services as part of the benefits package, but only by personally meeting the full cost. Access to health care would be much enhanced, it is argued, if qualified nurses or pharmacists could write prescriptions, at least for straightforward items.

To some extent views on the desirability of current regulatory outcomes are a matter of faith or belief. Those that accept allopathic medicine as the correct way to treat or to prevent illness will continue to believe that tight boundaries benefit the patient (clearly they certainly benefit the doctor). Advocates of alternative medicine cannot accept current outcomes of regulation. This battle will continue; in Chapter 7 we examine whether it is likely to constrain established members of the medical profession.

Part of the argument about access is, however, less dependent on beliefs or principles. It involves a debate about the desirability of allowing non-physicians who are accepted by doctors as (admittedly subservient) colleagues to treat and to prescribe. In all three countries the training of nurses, therapists, pharmacists and other 'paramedics' has become increasingly rigorous. Few now would agree that qualified nurses, for example, cannot be trusted to prescribe simple remedies for common illnesses. Indeed, in the UK and in the USA there are a number of experiments with the concept of 'nurse practitioners' to examine this argument. But until the boundaries are generally redrawn to take account of the professionalization of non-physician health carers, the outcome of regulation is to reduce access to some kinds of care which it is in the interests of patients to receive.

In Germany the outcome for patients is further affected by the balance of numbers between doctors and nurses. Alongside a German 'doctor glut' (over-supply) there exists a long-standing nursing shortage. This is because in recent years the pressure to contain costs in the German system has fallen much more heavily on nursing than on doctoring services.

Another aspect of competitive practices which has been subject to regulation is advertising. We saw earlier that in both US and UK governmental initiatives in recent years have made the profession's restrictions on advertising illegal, with varied results. The outcome of a ban on advertising has been, from the viewpoint of the patient, excessive secrecy about the qualifications, experience, range of services available, and levels of charges of physicians. Patients want *some* regulations to apply, to ensure that advertisements are honest and do not attack competitors but focus on the strengths of the advertiser. In the UK, for example, advertisements for opticians and for solicitors now often indicate new benefits such as discounts on eye tests or initial consultations at no charge, because advertising has enhanced competition. In America competition also ensures that both hospitals and doctors can widely advertise their facilities and skills.

Market structures

Two aspects of regulation are of particular concern to patients – the impact of referral systems, and the arrangements for clinical audit. In both instances we know that practice varies markedly between the three countries under review.

Referral systems in the UK and Germany ensure that local practice doctors are gatekeepers, with access to hospital care depending on their consent (some exceptions, like emergencies, apart). In the USA there are no regulations about referrals, and patient access to specialists is direct. In Germany, too, there is access to specialists who are in local practice: the domination of local practice by the all-purpose GP is unique to the UK.

Different regulatory outcomes are thus clear. Whether or not one of the three systems is best for patients is much less clear. In the UK, for example, it is a source of frustration to some that they can only see a specialist consultant after first convincing their GP of their need to do so (and waiting lists for consultant appointments adds to the frustration). On the other hand, the non-regulated open-access US approach results in no one doctor having any overall responsibility for the care of a patient, and no coordination of medical records, drug regimes and simultaneous care plans.

Similar complaints are heard in the German system: that the 'fee-for-service' payment system encourages duplication of tests and treatments by local practice doctors and hospitals; and the rigid separation between the two sectors means that coordination and patient record keeping are poor. The contrasting regulatory outcomes are interesting in their own right, but impossible to assess qualitatively in terms of their impact on patient care.

Clinical audit is somewhat easier to assess. The regulation of audit has been badly lacking. Neither self-audit, nor peer audit, nor external audit have been required as conditions of registration or licensing. Even in-service training to keep updated on medical developments has not been required in the UK or in a number of US states (in others re-registration at intervals is required and there are set minima for hours of training attended).

Self-regulation of standards, then, has historically failed to ensure that on-going clinical competence is assessed and the burden has fallen on disciplinary systems which, it was noted earlier, have also been limited in their impact and have commonly operated only in very extreme cases. Systematic medical audit seems to have to be initiated elsewhere than within the profession – in the UK by the state and in the USA by both the state and payers such as insurance companies and businesses. Even in Germany, however, the long-established system of scrutiny operated by teams of doctors employed by the insurance funds is concerned with economy rather than with clinical competence. In the case of doctors in local prac-tice, for instance, it involves scrutiny of their claims for payment under the fee-for-service system, and the questioning of those claims if they depart from an 'average' level. Recently this system has been strengthened, but in the search for cost containment rather than in the search for more clinical competence.

Belatedly, medical audit in the UK was finally introduced as part of the 1989–91 reforms of the NHS. Special funds are set aside by the Government. The regulatory approach centres entirely on the establishment of internal peer review, either within a hospital or within a locality in the case of GPs. US audit began in the early 1970s under Medicare legislation and has been much extended in the last decade by private-sector payers (business, insurers) who have been anxious to constrain costs by reducing the amount of 'unnecessary care' which is likely to be present in a health-care payment system based on incentives to treat through the fee-for-service principle.

In contrast to the proposed UK system of audit, in the USA there is external review. Indeed, in the private sector there are even specialized utilization review companies, employed by businesses to check that a care plan is necessary. The allegation has been made that in the UK, audit will be too cosy, and that quality assurance is best obtained by a more external review of treatments. It should, however, be recalled that the UK system of salaries and capitation fees does at least reduce the incentive to treat patients unnecessarily, so audit can focus much more than in the USA on the quality of needed care and in this way may not require such positive external policing of doctors.

The outcome of regulations about clinical audit is not reassuring for patients. The profession historically left a major gap which has been filled by schemes which can give only partial confidence that quality is assured. In the UK, the charge that audit is token, has no teeth and is an 'old pals act' can easily be laid, given the in-house basis of regulations. In the USA the main focus has been on quantity of care rather than quality, thus dealing with only half of the issue.

Pay

Patients want regulations which prevent them from being exploited financially: the desirable outcome is fair pay for the work undertaken. What constitutes 'fair pay' is a matter of judgement, but the question here is whether there are regulatory approaches designed to make such a judgement.

In the UK and Germany patients can be reasonably satisfied that regulations do ensure that judgements about pay are made collectively and by groups which include non-doctors as well as doctors. Systems of global budgets and negotiated fee or salary levels are in existence, as described in Chapter 5. And while in Germany the balance of power in these negotiations has tended to favour doctors, nevertheless a structure of regulation does exist.

By contrast, in the USA there has been until recently a regulatory gap and the outcome of non-regulation has been high fees, high incomes for doctors, and little in the way of redress for dissatisfied patients. Doctors have been able to charge their 'usual, customary and prevailing' fees, and to top-up any Medicare set fees by supplementary bills to the patient (except in only one or two states which have sought to ban this practice, with the result that many doctors there refused to treat Medicare patients). The new post-1992 federally initiated fee schedules may, however, lead to a more satisfactory outcome for patients, particularly if the private sector of health care also seeks to adopt them as a basis for payment.

In addition to the issue of levels of pay, a related second issue about doctors concerns the balance of incentives. In all three countries the focus has historically been on treating diagnosed illnesses. There have been poor financial rewards for doctors undertaking health promotion and illness-prevention activities, and epidemiology has been viewed by the leaders of the medical profession as of secondary importance. This can only change if self-regulation is replaced by government-led regulation, in this case of doctors' pay. There is limited activity in this field – in the UK, for example, GPs now receive additional income for reaching certain vaccination and screening targets and for running health promotion clinics, but the amounts are quite low, while in Germany reforms at the end of the 1980s also introduced incentives for screening and other preventive measures. In general, however, regulations will continue to centre on 'sickness treatment' whereas a desirable outcome for patients is the avoidance of illness.

Patients: overview

Regulation has not safeguarded patients or promoted patients' interests to the extent that the medical profession has often claimed. Regulation has traditionally centred on professional freedom and has curtailed both competition and external review. In particular, there has been little quality assurance and, in the USA, little control over doctors' incomes, which have remained extremely high since they received a fillip in the early years of Medicare and Medicaid. Indeed, despite several cost containment measures, and despite a rapid growth in the numbers of doctors in the 1970s, US physicians' real incomes have remained constant.

The lack of adequate quality assurance is a major weakness of traditional regulation of the medical profession by the medical profession. Inadequate provisions for disciplinary action, for clinical audit, and even for compulsory continuing education have become apparent in our study of medical regulation. Professional autonomy has been granted to an excessive degree, and this cannot be said to be an outcome which is in the interests of patients.

THE IMPACT OF REGULATION ON PAYERS

'Payers' and patients were once identical. Nowadays this is rarely true. Patients often pay something at the moment of treatment; and many patients pay a great deal towards the cost of health care, either via taxation or in health insurance contributions. But most of the cost of health-care is paid for by institutions: by governments, employers, insurance funds. The interests of these institutions may overlap with, but are not identical with those of patients.

Payers' interests are in one way simple: to obtain the most cost-effective medical care. All other things being equal, this suggests a regulatory strategy of cost minimization. But all other things rarely are equal, and only a little thought is required to see that cost containment bought at the expense of quality may not be in the long-term interests of payers.

Payers, then share some of the interests of patients, in particular their focus on quality assurance. But payers also are at odds with patients. Patients want treatment, and want the best possible treatment. Costs, to them, are secondary, partly because in most economically advanced countries there is a widespread expectation that doctors will solve perceived health problems, and partly because under insurance and NHS systems patients do not directly have to meet the full cost out of their own pockets. Hence there is a constant and never-ending series of disputes between patients and payers over entitlements to treatment. In the UK such disputes often revolve around waiting times or queues; in the USA around eligibility criteria, deductibles, co-payments and premium levels; in Germany about both the level of co-payments and the range of benefits claimable under insurance schemes. (These often spread well beyond the narrow area of medical care. In the late 1980s, for instance, one issue in Germany concerned whether patients could continue to claim the cost of taxis taking them from home for treatment. Medical politics often exploits these clashes, with doctors and patients forming coalitions to fight alleged rationing of health care imposed on them by payers.)

At the root of any examination of contemporary struggles over costs between doctors and patients lies one of the great debates of the 1980s – central both to public policy in general, and to health-care policy in particular. This argument is about the relative merits in principle of regulation and of competition. In both the USA and the UK the political system threw up leaders (Reagan, Thatcher) who were staunch supporters of markets and competition as mechanisms of control. Competition was advocated as a way of ensuring that customers obtained what they wanted, whereas regulation was viewed as a distortion of the workings of the market, usually in the interests of suppliers and against those of consumers, customers or patients.

The attempt by payers to use competition as a mechanism of control has in practice had limited success, even in the USA. Indeed, US health care 'is perhaps the most regulated industry in the US' (Levin, 1980, p. 1). To apply competition on a large scale would have needed a regulatory revolution – as would, indeed, have been required in the UK and Germany. Additionally, there are powerful arguments that health care is not a commodity which can simply be left to market forces, because markets have losers as well as winners and politicians have to intervene in support of losers – whether they be hospitals, or doctors, or patients – when life itself is at stake. Consequently the debate about markets has resulted only in piecemeal forays aimed at de-regulation; the main edifice of regulation has been retained. Indeed, so muddied has been the debate that regulation has actually been extended into new fields such as doctor payment schedules in the USA, and details of the work expected of self-employed GPs in the UK.

In Germany the failure to use market forces to shift more costs onto the shoulders of patients is one of the central puzzles of health-care reform in the 1980s. After the return of a (pro-market) Christian Democratic dominated Government in 1982 there were wide expectations of a Wende (change) in the direction of policy. But despite a steady stream of small measures restricting entitlements and expanding co-payments, there has been no substantial move in the direction of de-regulation in health-care policy. Indeed, in some respects regulation has been strengthened – for instance, by closer scrutiny of doctors' fee claims and by closer control over their drug prescribing practices.

Market entry

Payers want to ensure that there are sufficient numbers of doctors to avoid excessive scarcity leading to overcharging for services. In Germany and in the USA this has been achieved since 1960 through expansion in medical education to meet the growing need for doctors. In the UK, expansion of medical schools took place at a slower rate, partly because the main payer, government, was able to achieve a balance in the supply of doctors by regulating the flow of foreign medical graduates. They, in particular, have been used extensively to populate the less fashionable specialties such as psychiatry, geriatrics and – in the 1960s – general practice. This regulatory approach had a double dividend for government, in both avoiding the rapid expansion of expensive medical education and allowing doctors' salaries to be controlled through the introduction of substantial numbers of physicians with relatively modest financial aspirations.

From the payers' perspective, then, regulation of market entry has been extremely successful in the UK. The outcome is just the opposite in our two other countries. Both managed to over-expand their medical schools, and both have consequently reached a position close to one of doctor surplus. Of course, under a classical market this would lead to lower fees and salaries and not to additional costs, but in neither the USA nor Germany has that happened for the generality of doctors. Hence, both have more doctors per head of population than almost anywhere else, but doctor incomes which are amongst the highest.

US payers also experienced the unsuccessful regulation of market exit. Instead of systems of medical audit and licensing board discipline, the USA has relied far more on liability insurance and malpractice litigation in the courts to sort out clinical problems. This has been extremely costly. A Canadian obstetrician who moved to Baltimore, for example, reported that his annual malpractice insurance premium rose from $1000 dollars in Canada to $108 000, and this has actually to be met by payers. UK governments, too, are concerned about rising levels of litigation and higher judicial awards, and in both countries payers have recently been debating alternative systems styled 'no fault compensation' as a way towards containing such costs.

Medical incompetence in the USA has traditionally been viewed as a matter for each state. This has led to a major regulatory gap whereby any doctor disciplined or struck off could simply move to another state and seek registration there. This gap was finally plugged by Congress through legislation in 1986 and 1987 which both made such doctors ineligible for Medicare fees and established the National Practitioner Data Bank. However, an indication of the strength of medical interests is that this new piece of regulatory machinery does not have to be consulted by state licensing boards, though it does by hospitals. And no past reports are to be stored, so the Bank's disciplinary records begin only from 1989. The US attachment to pluralism, federalism and fragmentation of payer authority thus considerably diluted regulatory initiative.

Competitive practices

Much of the general argument about regulation in the 1980s in the UK, and the USA revolved around the notion that de-regulation could enhance competition, and that this was in the interests of both patients and payers. As we saw earlier, the USA led the way with a series of moves designed to promote competition under the federal Anti-Trust Laws: for instance, boycotts of alternative medicine and local fee-setting cartels of doctors were outlawed, and advertising was to be allowed. UK moves have been much more limited, and slower. It was only in 1990 that restrictions on advertising by GPs were eased, and the refusal of the Government as NHS payer to accept alternative therapies such as osteopathy remains absolute, with the full support of the profession. In addition, the UK and the German referral systems continue to reduce competition between doctors.

The outcome of these US and very recent UK attempts at de-regulation cannot be assessed precisely in terms of their impact on payers' costs. Indeed, health economists are deeply divided about the whole issue of medical competition and its cost consequences.

What is clear is that it is dangerous for payers to assume that if doctors face enhanced competition this will necessarily reduce costs. Externally, for example, osteopaths do not claim to treat more cheaply than orthopaedic surgeons – indeed a recent UK experiment indicated that the use of osteopaths by the NHS could result in more effective treatment of certain conditions, but at considerably higher costs. Internal competition through advertising is equally unlikely to reduce costs because patients respond favourably to signs of a high level of facilities and therefore of treatment, and are little concerned with the financial consequences. Hence advertisements are likely to stress the range of technology available rather than the modesty of the fees charged, and there is pressure on payers to meet the costs of state-of-the-art equipment and of skilled and extensive support teams working with the doctor.

In cost terms much more promising outcomes could stem from other areas of the regulation of competitive practices than these. The medical monopoly over the prescribing of drugs is one example. This has yet to be frontally tackled in the UK and the USA, but is being slowly eroded in Germany, where we saw earlier that the doctor–pharmacist boundary has become increasingly blurred. In the USA, the medical profession has quietly accepted some nurse prescribing in remote rural areas where access to a doctor is extremely difficult. In the UK, there have been one or two experiments which involve bending the rules rather than the outright delegation of prescribing responsibility to 'nurse practitioners', but the medical monopoly remains to all intents and purposes total. In addition, UK doctors have successfully retained their responsibility (in exchange for a separate fee each time) for verifying or refusing many welfare state benefits or entitlements such as invalidity benefit and mobility allowance.

If payers can move towards further de-regulation of some of these aspects of competitive (or, rather, non-competitive) practices, they can reasonably anticipate some cost savings. These might be in administrative overheads, where arguably unnecessary communication between pharmacist or nurse and doctor to obtain authorization for simple medications might be cut out, or in the substitution of less expensive labour, through nurses or social workers assessing eligibility for benefits.

Market structures

It is by now apparent that there are major differences between our three countries in the market structures within which doctors are organized. In the UK and Germany there is a clear distinction between hospital doctors and doctors in local practice, whereas in the USA, physicians provide care in both their main street offices and in hospitals where they have admitting rights. In the UK, local doctors are all-purpose general practitioners, whereas in the USA and Germany there are specialists outside the hospitals. UK and German referral systems for hospital care contrast with the US absence of such an approach. In the discussion on patients and regulation the variety of medical audit practices was revealed, with external review in the USA but peer group oversight only in the UK. US doctors can practice anywhere, and in Germany there have been few moves to regulate location but in the UK the Government has closely regulated this to equalize patient access to medical care. Finally, US doctors can and often do have financial interests in hospitals and pathology laboratories, whereas in the UK this only applies to the tiny private sector.

Not surprisingly these differences of market structures have a variable impact on payers. Furthermore, that impact or outcome is not necessarily dependent on regulation. Status and history, for example, can be important factors. German local practice doctors have a high status and consequently have historically commanded high incomes and been high cost physicians from the perspective of payers. UK GPs are, in contrast, a cheap option as traditionally the more ambitious doctors have sought hospital specialist posts. In the USA, surgeons have been the fashionable specialty, with consequences similar to the UK in terms of costs as the dwindling band of US 'family practitioners' have for decades commanded modest (relatively at any rate) incomes.

Regulation may challenge or may reinforce the cost consequences of status and history. In the USA, for instance, the introduction of utilization review by both the market sector (employers paying for benefits packages in particular) and by government, challenged the professional clinical autonomy of surgeons, and led to cost reductions through the investigation of allegedly unnecessary care. In sharp contrast, as we saw in the discussion of patients and regulation, the recent introduction of medical audit in the UK appears to be unconnected with cost and to offer little or no challenge to established interests as it is to be conducted locally and cosily through peer review. Indeed, in cost terms it is being funded by government through an additional earmarked budget running to several million pounds a year.

Many other UK regulatory approaches to market structures have also resulted in higher costs as the outcome. This is because the major UK payer, government, has sought to ensure reasonably equitable access to medical care, and to do this it has had to offer financial incentives to encourage doctors (and dentists and pharmacists) to practice in unpopular areas – remote rural counties and, the reverse, derelict and poverty-stricken inner cities. In terms of the global health budget the amounts are modest. Nevertheless they indicate that government as a cost-containing payer and government as a carer can face contradictory pressures.

US government has played little or no part in the regulation of physician ownership of health-care facilities, and regulations about this are entirely the responsibility of the profession. The AMA's ethical rules are quite clear – doctors must inform patients of any financial interests before recommending that patients utilize any such facilities. But the monitoring and policing of these rules has been lax, with considerable cost consequences for payers. A 1989 federal government study of Medicare patients revealed that one doctor in eight had ownership interests and that Medicare claims relating to patients referred by these physicians to 'their' facilities were staggeringly high. Such patients received 45 per cent more services than Medicare patients in general, but the AMA side-stepped government proposals for enhanced policing and disciplinary activity. In the UK, too, government has left it to the profession to regulate the private-sector activity of doctors, many of whom have ownership interests in the small private hospital sector, and increasingly in the rapidly growing private nursing home market. In Germany, doctor participation in hospital ownership is particularly marked in the field of convalescent sanatoria.

Pay

In contrast to the complexity of regulation of market structures, the regulatory outcome of doctors' pay is a good deal clearer, when viewed in cost terms, from the perspective of the payers. Again, history and status play their part, with the early introduction of national insurance in Germany and, from 1911, in the UK leading to negotiated fee levels. In contrast, it was not until the 1960s that US government became directly involved in health care and by then modern high-tech medicine was firmly established.

There is no doubt that the regulation of doctors' pay can in theory constrain costs, but it is equally clear that payers can have no guarantee that this will be the certain outcome of regulation. Outcomes are variable for two main reasons. First, the status of doctors may make it impossible to impose cost constraining regulations upon them against their will. Secondly, the payment system may make it difficult for regulators to control both price and volume.

In the USA, in particular, both these factors have worked to maintain high incomes for physicians and to minimize regulatory impact upon these incomes. The payment system of 'fee for service' continues to be predominant (there are few salaried doctors) and in itself it encourages activity – the more the doctor runs tests and offers treatment, the more he or she earns. The fragmentation of payers between employers, insurers, governments and individual citizens has prevented simultaneous regulatory activity over both fee levels and the volume of activities. Thus Medicare fees have commonly been topped-up by second bills to patients – one of many forms of cost-shunting practised in the USA – and by increasing the numbers of pre-treatment diagnostic tests undertaken.

In contrast to the USA, payers seem at first sight to benefit from regulation in the UK. The UK NHS operates through a global budget, an annual review of doctors' incomes, and a strong centralized political leadership seeking to minimize cost, and therefore tax, increases. Consequently pay rises are incremental, open (in aggregate) to public scrutiny, and largely unrelated to volume of activity. Indeed, salaried hospital doctors have no incentive to treat, and if GPs earn too much the amount is clawed back in later years in a way in which the US Government is seeking to copy. British doctors negotiated the right to undertake private work when the NHS was established, and some earn a lot from this, but globally private medicine is only a very small part of health care.

The regulation of pay in Germany sets up highly visible conflicts of interest between doctors and payers. The latter are, mainly, the insurance funds – and, eventually, their members who pay contributions. In the 'ambulatory' sector the conflict is visible in the negotiations to fix the global sum to be disbursed for treatment, which takes place between doctors' representatives and representatives of the insured. In the hospital sector the conflict is not with doctors themselves – who are largely salaried employees of hospitals – but with the institutions and their representatives.

In the past the balance of advantage, especially in the ambulatory sector, has been in favour of doctors. The insurance funds have lacked the unity to confront doctors over fee levels, and have lacked the organizational resources effectively to monitor the charging practices of doctors.

Payers – overview

Despite numerous forays, the outcome of regulation has, for payers, been generally disappointing. With the possible exception of the UK, doctors have maintained much of their financial autonomy and have been little affected in the pocket by regulation. Certainly a feature of the last 20 years has been their ability to maintain real incomes despite increasing concern in all countries about rising health-care costs. The status of doctors, and their political clout, has ensured that the bulk of cost containment is directed at other aspects of health care – in the USA at hospitals through the introduction of Diagnostic Related Groups; in the UK at 'management' and administrative overheads; in Germany at the patient by cost-sharing.

Payers, then, have found that regulation does not necessarily match up to their expectations, or result in outcomes reflecting their interests. In theory, regulation can control costs through enhancing competition and limiting incomes of doctors. In practice, the outcomes have more commonly been ones reinforcing existing medical monopolies, strengthening the demands of patients for more, and more expensive, medical care, and retaining or even raising existing income levels. The few examples which run counter to this have not managed to introduce, or get the profession to introduce, regulations which significantly constrain doctors.

CONCLUSIONS

Two points emerge strongly from our review of the outcomes of regulation. First, outcomes are variable as between countries. Secondly, outcomes are unpredictable.

Every aspect of regulation that we considered – supply, competitive practices, market structures, and pay – threw up variability. Doctors are plentiful in the USA and Germany but scarce in the UK. Behaviour and discipline are more tightly scrutinized in the UK than in USA. The medical monopoly *vis-à-vis* osteopaths remains in place in the UK, but not in the USA. The UK and Germany have referral systems; Germany and the USA allow specialists to practise locally. Pay is through the incentive-to-treat approach in the USA, where global budgets and salaries play little part; global budgets exist in Germany, but within the budget a fee-for-service system operates.

Unpredictability of regulation was also illustrated. Despite global budgets, usually thought to result in downward pressure on doctors' incomes, German physicians remain extremely well paid. Self-employed status and some item of service incentive payments have not made UK GPs more wealthy than their salaried hospital colleagues. Ethical codes about ownership of facilities have not deterred US doctors from referring patients at an alarming rate to services in which they have an interest.

Why have we found variable and unpredictable regulatory outcomes? Four factors seem to play a part in explaining these results – history; health-care systems; medical politics; and political coalitions. By history we mean the way in which regulation developed in each country. The UK was the early regulator, with state approval of professional self-regulation in the mid-nineteenth century. The strength of the BMA which resulted from the institution of the General Medical Council helped shape the organization of the profession before the end of the century. Hence the referral system and the medical monopoly, in particular, pre-dated active state involvement in health care. By contrast, in Germany the introduction of national insurance so quickly after the emergence of the nation-state predated nationally organized medicine and resulted in a fragmented, federal structure of separate medical organizations. Regulation in the USA came even later, but the early years of the twentieth century witnessed one vitally important development: in a fragmented political system there grew up in the American Medical Association a united national voice speaking on behalf of all physicians. The strength of the AMA lay precisely in its national unity, which it sought to develop initially through its own federal structure of 'closed shop' local societies, and later through accommodating the rise of specialties by altering its constitution in order to give them status and representation.

It would be natural to assume that health-care systems will affect regulatory outcomes. In Germany that is, in a sense, true in that the insurance system and the growth of state and self-regulation went hand-in-hand. But in the UK and the USA, today's health-care systems are relatively recent creations. By the time US government became involved in health care in the 1960s, the regulatory approach which gave doctors enormous influence over all aspects of medicine was in place. Consequently the contemporary system remains in many respects unchanged. Regulatory outcomes have affected the supply of doctors, and have outlawed monopoly behaviour, though in the latter case with few practical consequences. The structure of physician pay is currently in the limelight, but until at least the early 1990s medical power over market structures, income, and many aspects of licensing, discipline and competitive practices has not been effectively challenged.

The UK NHS built on the earlier 1911 insurance system, but altered it dramatically when the state assumed direct control of hospital provision. However the new system allowed doctors to either continue as self-employed or, in the case of hospitals, to top-up their salaries. Despite state near-monopoly, clinical audit was not regulated until 1990 and competitive practices and market structures were little altered. Pay has been a political issue from time to time, with new regulations based on independent review introduced in the late 1960s. In terms of outcomes, however, doctors' pay in real terms or relative to national average pay has remained remarkably constant: if there has been a regulatory outcome it has been stability. As this same stability was found in both Germany and the USA, it is difficult to offer the health-care system as a positive factor influencing outcomes.

Medical politics are a third potential influence on regulatory outcomes. Organizationally, doctors are strong in the USA and in the UK, with national associations which have a political monopoly to all intents and purposes. In Germany there is superficially organizational fragmentation, with organizations functioning most effectively at the level of Länder. But since other actors are even more fragmented, and since the ruling groups in doctors' organizations are joined in well-connected networks, the political muscle of physicians remains formidable. And in all three countries, doctors derive power from their high status. As respected members of the community and, perhaps more important, as essential members, their voices carry great weight. Consequently, political attacks on the tradition of professional self-regulation can only be sustained by very tough politicians. In truth, politicians have little to gain from confronting doctors, and possibly have many votes to lose. Debates in all three countries about cost containment, perhaps *the* single most important issue in the 1980s, have illustrated very well the power of medical politics. US politicians focused on hospitals, UK ministers on management systems. Only when the UK Government faced continued crises centring on waiting times did it seek to regulate doctors directly, and in 1989–91, a battle ensued with the profession continually influencing public opinion into believing that the Government's policies might not work. And as soon as the new regulatory machinery was in place, a new minister sought peace talks and offered concessions to the doctors in general practice through relaxing the controls imposed upon them.

Finally, political coalition-forming can influence the extent and outcome of medical regulation. In this chapter we have analysed outcomes from the three standpoints of doctors, patients and payers. On certain issues, doctors and patients form a powerful potential political alliance. They share interests in access to medical treatment, and in the quantity of care available – both issues which pressurize payers to spend more money. So successful have these pressures been that rising costs emerged by the 1980s as a crucial issue in all three countries. By the 1990s, however, there was little evidence of effective cost containment, with spending continuing to outstrip inflation and increasing as a proportion of Gross National Product. In short, the doctor–patient coalition remained in the driving seat, seemingly almost immune from any regulatory activity designed to curtail the quantity of medical intervention.

The quality issue is based on a rather different coalition. This time patients and payers share interests, the first because their health is at stake and the second because they ultimately pick up the bill for any unnecessary or unskilled treatment. Hence in the USA, Utilization Review (UR) has been introduced successfully, and doctors now expect their work to be externally checked. What is slightly odd is the nature of UK regulation – with patients and payers seeming to have united views under an NHS system, early regulation on quality might have been expected, but did not happen.

Lastly, a patient–payer coalition on costs is more difficult to obtain because it depends on patients viewing the issue as insurance contributors or as taxpayers rather than as sick people in need of medical services, and the coalition is always liable to collapse because most citizens cannot continue, when ill, to take the taxpayer viewpoint. Hence doctors are able to exploit their unity with their patients, and the institutional payers are left isolated, and even labelled as 'uncaring' as they seek to tackle rising bills.

History, health-care systems, medical politics and different political coalitions all help explain the variety of regulatory outcomes found earlier in this chapter. In particular, they account for the continuing strength of doctors in all three countries. Self-regulation remains the norm, and state regulation is frequently fairly benign in its design, its implementation, or both. In essence, doctors have survived the introduction of large-scale governmental involvement in health care and the contemporary debate about rising costs, if not unscathed then certainly in pretty good health. That they have been on the defensive for many decades is inevitable, given these developments. Whether or not they have been, as they often claim, in decline is much less clear from the evidence offered above on regulatory outcomes. It is to this question of professional decline that we now turn.

FURTHER READING

An ambitious cross-national comparison of the impact of regulatory changes on doctors is in chapter 3 of Heidenheimer *et al.* (1990). Alongside it, see Harrison and Schulz's Anglo-American comparison of contrasts and convergence in Freddi and Björkman (1989) and also Wilsford (1991) – in chapter 10 he extends his study of the USA and France to embrace the UK and Germany (and Canada and Japan), concluding that battles between doctors and governments will remain a universal feature of health-care policy-making. One aspect of such battles relates to the introduction of the rationing of health care – on this, see Blank (1988); and the fascinating detailed comparative examination of the availability of ten medical procedures in the UK and the USA by Aaron and Schwartz (1984).

The debate about the possibility of over-doctoring through the expansion of medical schools is assessed by Weiner (1989). The disciplinary record of US licensing boards is found to be both patchy and generally weak by Schwartz and Mendelson (1989).

For Anglo-American comparisons look at Pollitt (1990) on the introduction of new quality-control systems in the 1980s; at Klein (1981) who argues that UK fixed budgets enable doctors to experience clinical freedom much more than do US doctors, and at Wood (1991) and Hiatt (1987) on attempts at cost-containment policies and physician responses to such moves. Baumol (1988) argues that US doctors remain able to side-step cost-containment measures and have maintained their real incomes as a result – and OECD (1990) shows their incomes to be among the highest in the world. Mechanic (1985) sees US patients as pliant, and concludes that any serious threats to physician autonomy have to come from elsewhere – from hospital chains, third-party payers or governments. Two US physicians, Grumbach and Bodenheimer (1990) foresee continued 'discomfort' and reduced clinical freedom as a result of cost-containment policies.

Studies of the impact of German regulation in the English language are rare. Moran (1990) looks at the question of doctor supply, and also at the main institutional payers, the insurance funds. Webber (1991) has some discussion of costs, as has the Deutsche Bundesbank (1991). A great deal can be gleaned about outcomes by looking closely at the comparative statistics on health-care systems produced by the Organization for Economic Co-operation and Development (OECD, 1985, 1987, 1990). Alber (1991) uses this data source to 'set' the German system in comparative perspective.

In the German language, Baier (1988) has produced a highly critical study of the impact of the modern organization of professional medicine; from a different position Scholmer (1984) has criticized the commercial organization of the profession. 'Impact' discussions in Germany have, apart from the previously mentioned examination of pay levels, focused mostly on issues of inequality. There are studies of the unequal distribution of doctors in Schardt and Wendt (1987) and in Wendt (1985). There are also studies of the unequal burdens imposed by the structure of the insurance funds, in Cyffka (1988) and Pick and Plein (1989).

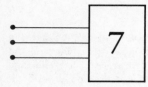

DOCTORS IN DECLINE?

INTRODUCTION

Doctors are one of the most important interests in the modern state. This importance springs from a range of well-known factors. In part it is the result of the key functions performed for society by the medical profession. Health is a highly valued condition in all societies, and in modern societies doctors have been seen as the main agents in ensuring good health. But the doctor's role in medical care and assessment has gone beyond the treatment of the sick. As Stone (1984) has shown, one of the chief grounds for access to welfare help from the modern state is 'disability' – demonstration that an individual is unable for reasons of physical or mental handicap to make a living by competing in the labour market. And almost universally doctors are central to the process by which claimants are certified as unfit – either as short-term sick or as long-term disabled. Thus the social functions of the doctor go well beyond the obvious, important sphere of health care; doctors are a key profession in the functioning of modern welfare states.

Any occupational group which performs key social functions, as does the medical profession, is likely to enjoy a position of prestige and influence with modern governments. But physicians have further strengthened their position by the way they have organized. As we have seen in earlier chapters in the three very different health-care systems of the USA, UK and Germany, the medical profession shows striking common patterns of organization. In all three countries there are powerful bodies which exercise significant, if varying, control over key matters like entry, pay and competition.

It is small wonder, in the light of all this, that doctors acquired the reputation as a uniquely powerful group in the modern state. But as we saw in Chapter 2 there have, in recent years, been some observers who believe that this power is in decline. The purpose of this concluding chapter is to ask how far the evidence discussed in the preceding chapters supports this view. First of all we look at our three countries in turn, and then we discuss the wider implications of the evidence. Of course the phrase 'doctors in decline' suggests something very comprehensive. We could answer that question by reference to a whole range of factors: the most obvious include the power of doctors over patients, and the ability of doctors to extract rewards from the market. 'Decline' is also a temporal notion; it conveys a change in condition between two periods. Thus any statements about decline ought, if possible to specify the time period which is being discussed.

In what follows, the 'decline' examined is fairly narrow. The focus of this book has been regulation – and, in particular, the nature of the relationships between doctors and the state in the regulatory process. In raising the question of 'doctors in decline', therefore, we ask whether the relationship between doctors and the state has changed, and how far this change, insofar as it has occurred, has tilted control of regulation away from the doctor. Of course put in this bald way many important questions are begged. Can we speak of 'the state' as a single institution impacting on doctors in a uniform way? Even if the state intervenes in a coherent manner, is it to be expected, given the known divisions within the medical profession, that all doctors will be affected in the same way? These questions are, however, best tackled in the examination of the particular countries, precisely because the structure of the state, the structure of the medical profession and the content of regulation all vary from country to country. In the final section we ask what has happened, overall, to the balance between the doctor and the state.

GERMANY

There have been two key periods in the regulatory history of the medical profession in Germany: a few years spanning the end of the Weimar Republic and the Nazi seizure of power in the 1930s; and a second period, the decade following the end of the Second World War.

In the reforms of the 1930s the medical profession – and especially that part of it in local practice – secured a highly favourable regulatory bargain with the state. It is from this period that some of the key modern features of regulation date: the confirmation of the chambers as the most important regulatory institutions for the individual doctor; the exclusion of the health insurance funds from any significant role in employing doctors or in otherwise providing medical services; and the rise of the Insurance Doctors' Associations as both bargainers about payment with the insurance funds and as administrators of the payment system. The significance of the decade after the end of the Second World War is that, following a brief period when it seemed possible that Germany might adopt a health-care system in which government played the sort of direct role characteristic of the National Health Service in the UK, the patterns of the 1930s were restored: the insurance funds were confirmed as paymasters, but the doctors' control over the provision of health care was also restored, as was the central place of their institutions, the Insurance Doctors' Associations.

The years after 1955 were probably the height of doctors' power in Germany. They successfully repulsed an attempt at reform in the late 1950s (described in Webber, 1988). The German economy enjoyed unprecedented prosperity and this paid for a continuing expansion of the health-care budget. Perhaps the only significant defeat suffered by doctors occurred with the constitutional court's decision (see Chapter 5) striking down the rule limiting membership of Insurance Doctors' Associations to a fixed ratio of population. But even this was less a case of defeat at the hands of the state, and more a case of one group of doctors winning a victory at the expense of another: it reflected the demands of hospital doctors, with ambitions to enter medical practice, not to be shut out by those already established as local practitioners.

The world of health care in Germany for the last 15 years or so has been very different from the world of plenty that prevailed in the 1950 and 1960. After the mid-1970s Germany, like most other advanced capitalist economies, experienced significant economic difficulties. This coincided with a growing perception that the rate of growth in health-care spending sustained in the previous couple of decades could not continue. From the mid-1970s, therefore, Germany, like most other health-care systems, entered an era when 'cost containment' was the dominant theme of policy debates. Since doctors are the chief agents of costs in the health-care system – either through their own fees and salaries or through the treatment they prescribe – the search for cost containment has impinged on the medical profession. How far this has seriously constrained the regulatory freedom of doctors is, however, a matter of some uncertainty.

There are indeed some signs that the regulatory freedom of doctors has been constrained. There is undoubtedly greater attention paid to the economic behaviour of doctors by ministers at both federal and state level. Until the late 1980s, this interest had little effect on the actual substance of regulation. The legislation passed at the end of that decade, however, may represent a significant incursion by the state. In the name of cost containment the law, as we saw earlier, has intruded on the prescribing habits of doctors, empowering pharmacists to alter their prescriptions if they prescribe drugs for which, in the pharmacist's judgement, there exists a cheaper equivalent alternative.

Legislation at the end of the 1980s also significantly changed the balance of roles inside the Insurance Doctors' Associations. The fact that since the 1930s the Associations were central to the administration of the payment system always gave them a mixed character. On the one hand they are doctors' organizations – dominated by a key section of the profession, and defending its interests. On the other hand, as administrators of the payment system for ambulatory care they have had a 'control' function – the duty of scrutinizing doctors to prevent illegitimate or fraudulent claims. For most of their history this control function was performed in a very limited way, but at the end of the 1980s, in the name of cost containment, it was markedly strengthened. For instance, both the proportion of doctors 'audited', and the range of their activities so audited, significantly widened. Thus one of the key organizations in the life of the ambulatory doctor seems to be changing its character – from an organization that primarily defended physicians' interests to one which controls the working life of the doctor.

Against this picture of German doctors increasingly hemmed in by the state should be set four factors which suggest that doctor autonomy from the state remains very great. First, the state in Germany is in general an unlikely agent of tight control. The federal government in Bonn does not have either the administrative resources or the constitutional power to intervene in a health-care system whose institutions are fragmented into the separate Länder and into a wide range of private and semi-public bodies. This observation is strengthened, second, by what happened to policy in the 1980s. The return of the Christian Democrats to office as the main governing party in Bonn in 1982 was hailed as the start of a Wende – a major turning point in policy which would take Germany sharply in the direction of an economy where market forces operated more strongly. One of the puzzles of German politics generally in the 1980s is why that Wende failed to materialize, whereas it did in, for example, the UK and the USA. And in the case of health care, observers have also noted the failure to push through radical changes in the decade. In brief, the course of public policy in the decade does not suggest a dramatic curtailment by the state of doctors' power.

A third reason for stressing the continuing freedom of doctors from state intervention is that in the one area where there does seem to be taking place a noticeable curtailment of doctors' freedom – in the growth of the control functions of the Insurance Doctors' Associations – the Associations nevertheless remain firmly under the control of the doctors themselves. Indeed, in general, the really effective challenge to the doctors comes, not from the state, but from the payers – who in Germany, as we know, are represented by the autonomous Insurance Funds. In other words, insofar as the balance of power in the health-care system is shifting it is shifting, not from the doctor to the state, but from the doctor to the payer.

A fourth and final reason for believing that the power and autonomy of German doctors has not been seriously damaged concerns the impact of German re-unification. The precise shape of the system being constructed in the territories of the previous German Democratic Republic is still unclear, but it is certain that it will result in a pattern of regulation close to that of the previous Federal Republic, and very unlike that practised under the former Communist regime. And the most striking feature of the medical profession under Communism was its low independence and prestige. Doctors were poorly paid, and enjoyed little of the status and independence accorded the free professions in local practice in West Germany. In other words, re-unification has destroyed a system where the medical profession was weak, and is replacing it by one where the medical profession is strong.

In summary, we can say that of our three cases, Germany emerges as the country where the power of doctors has retreated least in recent years.

USA

We saw in Chapter 3 that the mid-1960s form a clear dividing point in US medical history. At that time government became heavily involved, for the first time, in both the scale of medical education and in the provision of access to care for the elderly and poor. A decade later witnessed more state activity with the introduction of Peer Review Organizations to check on the actions of individual doctors, and with the series of Anti-Trust court hearings designed to make doctors compete more openly both with other doctors and with alternative providers of care such as chiropractors.

This increased government activity ran alongside a change in the owner-ship of many hospitals, and the rise of the 'for-profit' hospital chains. Medicine was allegedly becoming corporatized and bureaucratized, and many academic observers began to talk of the 'deprofessionalization' and even the 'proletarianization' of doctors. The 1960s were seen as a benchmark with any golden age of medicine having preceded the events of that decade.

Our analysis of regulation does not easily fit into this thesis of rapidly declining professional autonomy, certainly not across the board. In particular, we found the 1960s to have been a decade of great opportunity for US doctors to enhance their incomes, and they took it. The Medicare and Medicaid programmes proved to be a 'bonanza'.

US doctors continue to operate as largely self-employed, solo practitioners. Though hospitals do employ salaried physicians, the key feature of admitting rights for doctors with offices outside the hospital remains – a form of referral to oneself not known in either Germany or the UK. Indeed, the side-stepping by hospitals of some of the impact of Diagnostic Related Group (DRG) fixed fees actually strengthened this feature by encouraging physicians to undertake more of the pre-operative diagnostic tests outside the hospital: the bond between a physician and the hospitals to which he or she admits thus remains strong. The reduced need for hospitalization as, universally, day surgery and drug regimes reduce both admissions and length of stay further strengthen the position of the US physician. Hospitals compete for patients, and hence for physicians to take up admitting rights with them.

Why, then, do US doctors and their professional (colleges) and pressure group (AMA) organizations so frequently complain about their declining autonomy? First, they complain because they are politicians. Wearing their political hats they seek to maximize their professional freedom, their incomes, their social status, and their quality of life. This is perfectly natural and perfectly reasonable – it is exactly what any political pressure group does. It means that any proposal to change the existing regulatory system will be instantly analysed publicly in terms of the potential impact on the status and freedom of the doctor, while any analysis of opportunities to improve pay, status or autonomy remains private. Consequently US medical politics appears to be largely negative politics, and medical politicians seem to be seeking to defend the *status quo* rather than to want to initiate change. Underneath this veneer, of course, doctors actually have privately been happy to accept many changes – not least the improved access to care which began in the 1950s with the large-scale growth of employment-related insurance schemes and continued in the 1960s with Medicare and Medicaid. After all, better access to care for the American people meant more work for doctors. Furthermore, the profession has been extremely successful in managing to maintain the system of doctor-determined 'fee-for-service' payment which preceded private and state insurance schemes.

Second, US doctors complain because they have been experiencing some declining autonomy alongside the growth in incomes and continuity, or even improvement, in status *vis-à-vis* hospitals. In particular they have had no option but to accept greater bureaucratization, some over-supply, the rise of 'managed care', and the widespread introduction of Utilization Review.

Once the patient is not the payer, form-filling is inevitable. The 'cost' of greater access, through private insurance, usually linked to employment, and through government schemes of Medicare and Medicaid, is bureaucracy. Doctors thus require administrative support staff on a scale unimaginable 50 years ago, when the vast majority of patients simply paid up there and then. And there is uncertainty – will the bill be paid in full without query? When will the payment arrive? American doctors have become businessmen, but it is not at all clear that this increased bureaucracy has, *on its own*, reduced their professional freedom.

We have already seen that in many urban areas there is now a very large supply of doctors. This is a direct consequence of federal decisions back in the 1960s to encourage the rapid expansion of medical schools in the light of the then shortage of US-trained physicians and the heavy dependence on immigrant doctors. The replacement of what had traditionally been professional self-regulation of medical education by direct state regulation has thus not been in the narrow interests of doctors, who, in many urban areas of over-supply, are now having to compete fairly aggressively for patients. In terms of the medical tradition of high social status, this is considered by some physicians to be demeaning, and the AMA fought hard against the 1970s and 1980's Anti-Trust moves.

The rise of 'managed care' and of utilization review are perhaps the greatest threats to the profession. Managed care is another manifestation of competition and de-regulation, and it developed in the 1970s as a response to the greatest crisis confronting US health care – exploding costs. The Nixon Administration was the first to encourage the growth of Health Maintenance Organizations (HMOs), which pose a direct threat to the profession in that they often employ salaried physicians, and work on the basis of a fixed annual charge (or capitation fee) for all care, rather than on the much-valued (by doctors) traditional fee for service. HMOs have thus had no incentive to treat patients and every incentive to promote preventive services, with the consequence that they have reduced costs.

Utilization Review (UR), also a response to the cost explosion of the late 1960s, much more directly impacts on almost every US doctor. Reviewers have questioned the need for many treatments and physicians can expect to have their medical patient records examined at any time. This direct challenge to the individual clinical autonomy of US doctors has reduced their freedom to diagnose and treat patients in a way not (yet) experienced in either Germany or the UK. UR, a growth industry since the early 1970s and now widely used by insurance companies and by large employers anxious to contain costs, lies at the heart of the complaint by US doctors that their professional freedom has been eroded.

But the cost explosion in the USA has continued, despite HMOs and despite UR. Doctors now face yet another challenge, and one which threatens their traditional fee-for-service incomes. For Medicare there are to be fixed fee schedules, phased in over the four years 1992–5. As with UR, the private-sector payers (insurance companies and employers) will undoubtedly adopt a similar approach if the fee schedules do prove to contain costs by reducing doctors' incentives to provide financially lucrative and expensive surgical procedures in particular.

The evidence from the USA about the extent of doctors' decline is, it seems, contradictory. Certainly their *modus operandi* has changed this last 30 years, and they have become in effect small businesses running an office full of high-tech equipment and of practice management staff. They first had to respond to major changes in access to health care – insurance and governmental schemes which have separated the patient from the payer. They then were confronted by early cost-containment policies, some of which focused on clinical autonomy. Finally, they have had to adjust to the 1980s' moves to further control costs through fixed hospital, and now physician, fees.

Doctors in the USA appear to have adjusted successfully to these regulatory changes. Their income status has actually risen over this 30-year period, and they have not suffered unduly from competition from alternative providers of health care. They collectively continue to lay down many standards of professional behaviour, as was seen in Chapter 4, and their national Association remains an outstanding example of a powerful pressure group. Their self-employed status has very largely been retained, and they are perhaps more able than ever to 'call the shots' in their relationships with hospitals which desperately seek patients.

In short, the regulatory machinery, outputs and outcomes have changed, as we saw in Chapters 4 to 6, and the social and economic context within which doctors work has changed. But it is essential that we do not equate change with decline, for change has brought US doctors opportunities to better themselves as well as some additional burdens. The post-War revolution inevitably did not leave medicine untouched, nor unscathed, but neither did it challenge the key role that physicians play in American society and health care. Indeed, some say that the greatest burden has been imposed on US physicians not by insurance companies, big business or government, but by individual patients. Patients increasingly expect and demand a perfect outcome to their treatment, and have increasingly had recourse to the courts if their expectations are not fulfilled. The spate of 'malpractice' cases has probably made many doctors – surgeons and obstetricians in particular – more cautious of offering diagnosis and treatment than have the activities of the Utilization Reviewers. In that sense, US medicine has seen the rise of patient power as much as regulator power.

UK

The introduction of the National Health Service (NHS) in 1948, and its overhaul in 1989–91, have been key events affecting the role, status and professional freedom of all UK doctors. UK general practitioners, in addition, were also much affected by the 1911 introduction of national health insurance and by the 1965 GPs' Charter. Government played a central role as policy initiator in each case, and government in the UK is directly responsible for the provision of almost all health care. State provision of social care through the post-1945 welfare state also involves doctors – they are key gatekeepers because claimants of many social security benefits need a medical examination as a crucial part of the process of determining eligibility.

Given this central role of government it is perhaps surprising that the medical profession in the UK has continued to be either self-regulatory or heavily involved in state-led regulation. The 1948 and 1989–91 reforms have been seen as exceptional, in that in both instances regulation was imposed on unwilling doctors: more common is a situation where government negotiates with the profession and seeks common ground and consensus agreements. Because of this convention of negotiated agreement, the British Medical Association has been much more willing than its US sister organization to accept direct governmental involvement in the funding of medical schools, in decisions about doctors' pay, and even in the introduction of a 'limited list' of drugs which cannot be prescribed. (In 1985 the 'limited list' removed the right of GPs to prescribe under the NHS some 200 drugs where either the medical benefits were unclear or there was felt to be a suitable, normally cheaper, alternative.) For political reasons there was an airing of opposition to the regulation of pay and prescribing, but the pragmatic UK profession was always prepared to negotiate.

The high-water mark of UK medicine was probably in the late 1960s. In that era of what has often been labelled 'consensus politics' the prevailing wisdom was that experts knew best. Hence health care should be left to doctors. There was broad agreement across the main political parties about the existence of the welfare state, including the NHS, and a general belief that steady growth would continue to allow poverty to be reduced and health to be improved. While the costs of the NHS, the pay of doctors, and the role and status of general practitioners had all at one time been extremely contentious political issues, by 1965 negotiated agreements between the BMA and the government had been reached on each of these three. Crucially for the doctors, the agreed independent Remuneration Board appeared to offer a guarantee of an acceptable rate of income increase.

Any era of tranquillity was short-lived. The oil crisis of 1973 and the Government's NHS reforms of 1974 both removed stability and presaged the introduction of a more assertive and more regulatory governmental attitude towards medicine. Cost containment quickly reached the top of the health agenda, and has in effect stayed there ever since, as successive Labour (1974–9) and Conservative Governments have sought to exert some control over public expenditure.

Government 'solutions' to the problem of steadily increasing NHS costs have broadly been of two types. The first, the encouragement of greater use of private medicine through such policies as tax incentives, has not much affected doctors' freedoms. Indeed, the expansion of private medicine has frequently been to the benefit of doctors, as a fundamental agreement on the introduction of the NHS in 1948 was that they could continue to earn from private practice even while working technically full time for the NHS (see Chapter 3).

For hospital doctors the important policy thrust has stemmed from the introduction of managers and management teams within the NHS, and the search for 'efficiency'. The pace of change has been constant. In 1974 a system of 'consensus management' involved a 'team' including an administrator, a treasurer, a nurse and two doctors; a decade later this alleged consensus was replaced by the industrial concept of a General Manager; in 1989–91 even more fundamentally the roles of purchaser of care and provider were separated. Within only 17 years, doctors' status had been reduced from playing a central role in a team determining the pattern of hospital services in a locality to part of a group of health-care workers within an organization which had the task of providing care in accordance with contract specifications negotiated with a separate, purchasing health authority which was making hospitals compete with each other for contracts. During that period, not only General Managers (several from industry and the armed forces), but also value-for-money accountants and auditors arrived on the scene, and the Audit Commission (created by statute in 1983) began to publish reports which sharply impinged on the traditional clinical freedom of hospital doctors. In 1990, for example, the Commission criticized the failure of many surgeons to undertake what it considered to be a reasonable level of day surgery. Finally, the 1948 agreement to senior consultants receiving large bonuses determined secretly by doctor-only committees was amended: General Managers are now members of these committees.

General practitioners at first seemed exempt from the main thrust of cost-containment policy, with the notable exception of the introduction of a limited list of drugs which could be prescribed under the NHS. Though imposed, the list was actually negotiated and the boundaries of the profession held firm in that no powers were given to pharmacists to substitute cheaper equivalent drugs. This contrasts with the position not only in Germany (see above) but also in many UK NHS hospitals where hospital pharmacists are instructed by non-medical managers to dispense the generic or cheaper alternative to brand-named drugs.

The 1989–91 reforms, however, impinged sharply on several of the traditional areas of freedom of GPs. A new contract containing a more detailed specification of their work than ever before was imposed upon them – after a negotiated settlement, reluctantly agreed by BMA spokesmen, was rejected by the rank-and-file doctors. The appointed body locally responsible for monitoring the contract – the Family Health Services Authority (FHSA) – was strengthened, including the appointment of a General Manager, and instructed to manage GPs positively rather than merely to pay them. And the Government indicated that it expected all GPs to be involved in Medical Audit, earmarking funds to meet the costs and ordering the local appointment of doctor-led Audit Committees. This entry into Audit applied also to hospital doctors and, at least initially, was officially termed educative, non-threatening peer review with no involvement of non-doctors. Whether all this remains the case only time can tell.

This brief chronicle of events in 1989–91 may suggest another watershed, with doctors emerging from the process largely deprofessionalized. Certainly many UK doctors will see the reforms as an attack on their professional status, and there is little difficulty in amassing some quite convincing evidence that state regulation has taken over from self-regulation. But any political argument such as the one which took place between the Government and the medical profession in the UK between 1989 and 1991 is inevitably a mixture of rhetoric and reality. The heavy rhetoric of the debate was well illustrated by a BMA poster campaign directed against the then Secretary of State – *What Do You Call a Man Who Refuses to Listen to the Doctor's Advice? Kenneth Clarke* – a campaign reflecting the BMA's annoyance at a government prepared to impose without normal negotiations what seemed to be radical reforms of both the hospital and the GP services.

The reality is that doctors are now to be made more accountable, in both a financial and a non-financial sense, for their actions. GPs, for example, have to produce annual reports which *inter alia*, give data on their patterns of consultations and referrals. They are now expected to work within an indicative budget (not quite a cash limit, though cash control is the Government's aim) for prescribing costs, and a cash limit for assistance with their staffing and computer costs. They have genuine concerns that the new purchasing health authorities may limit their traditional freedom to refer patients to any hospital consultant in the UK. At the hospital level the reforms involve detailed costings of all activities. For the first time ever it will be known how much a particular episode of treatment actually costs in every hospital. Given the centrality of cost containment and the top–down imposition of fixed budgets within which the purchasing authority must operate, hospital doctors naturally fear that the pressure will be on to provide the cheapest possible service, with quality a secondary consideration. They believe, genuinely, that their ability to do what is best for the patient will be overridden by the demands of the accountants.

This all looks like very convincing evidence of doctors in decline in the UK following the 1989–91 reforms. But we must not forget that many said very much the same type of thing in the immediate post-1948 period, and in 1911. It is important not to over-respond to these three unique cases of a breakdown in relations between the profession and government. It is also important to remember that after both 1911 and 1948 normal relations were resumed fairly quickly, and the worst-case scenarios of the pessimists never did materialize.

History may well repeat itself. The 1989–91 reforms were barely on the statute book before a new Secretary of State showed signs of holding out an olive branch to the BMA. Within months negotiated agreements were once again being reached, this time on issues such as referral rights of GPs and waiting list arrangements in hospitals to ensure that all patients received equitable treatment (some were being referred to a hospital by the few GPs who were 'Fundholders', and who themselves could purchase from their own budget any necessary care for their patients, regardless of local purchasing authority policy, thus seemingly being in a position to jump the queue and create a two-tier health service).

Finally, the 1989–91 reforms were less than comprehensive. UK doctors retain the self-regulation of market entry and discipline exercised by the General Medical Council (see Chapter 4) and they still do not have to be re-accredited periodically in order to remain registered. Their ability to work for both the public and the private sectors; the self-employed status of GPs; the strict separation of hospital and general practice activity; the regulation of geographical distribution through hospital budgets and Medical Practices Committee decisions; and a great deal of clinical freedom (perhaps now more collective through the new Medical Audit Committees, but still entirely professionally organized, unlike the US example of Utilization Review): all remain scarcely if at all changed. Furthermore, in one key respect they retain a superior professional status to their German and US colleagues: the boundaries of the profession continue to hold secure, with virtually no intrusion by pharmacists or nurse prescribers, or by osteopaths, chiropractors or other providers of 'alternative medicine'. The state continues to recognize allopathic medicine as a legitimate mono-poly, just as it did when it passed the 1858 Act. The very existence of the NHS thus actually strengthens the status of doctors by severely restricting the ability of alternative providers to enter the market successfully.

CONCLUSION: DOCTORS, REGULATION AND THE STATE

The experience of the three countries examined here – the USA, the UK and Germany – shows that there is a complicated mixture of common patterns and national peculiarities in the connections between doctors, regulation and the state. The patterns might be summarized under the headings 'power and pressure': everywhere doctors have power; but everywhere they are under pressure.

In all three countries doctors enjoy, and have for a long time enjoyed, great power. The roots of this power lie in the regulatory systems. All three have long practised some variety of self-regulation. The exact balance between independent self-regulation and state-licensed self-regulation varies, but the most striking feature is the degree to which doctors and their institutions are able to exercise control over entry to the profession, over its organization, over the degree of competition for patients, and over payment systems. In all three countries, doctors are influential and well-organized lobbyists. But their greatest influence lies less in their overt interventions in politics, and more in the way their everyday influence in regulation shapes outcomes.

But this common experience of power has gone alongside another common experience in recent years – doctors are everywhere under pressure. The sources of this pressure are various. They firstly come from the changing organization of the job market. At the turn of the century doctors were the most numerous group in health care; now they are a minority alongside nurses and a whole range of other medical occupations. In America, for example, physicians made up two-thirds of all health-care professionals in 1900, but less than ten per cent by 1980 (Levin, 1980, p. 88). The archetypical free professional in medicine is the doctor working independently in solo practice. Everywhere this figure is becoming less common: doctors are working in group practices, in hospitals, and for institutional 'suppliers' of health care like US Health Maintenance Organizations. Of course there is no intrinsic reason why doctors working in organizations should not be powerful. But the decline of the solo practitioner has coincided with alterations in the economic climate of medical practice. In all three countries – and in many more – the last two decades have been dominated by the struggle to contain the costs of health care. And since doctors are both a major cost themselves, and by their clinical decisions are major determiners and allocators of cost throughout health-care systems, those concerned to contain costs have increasingly turned their attention to the working practices of physicians.

It might be imagined that the inevitable result of these pressures would be a universal growth in state control: a shift away from independence to more state-directed forms of regulation, either through stricter state control over self-regulatory institutions or via the assumption of direct state responsibility. In practice, three sets of factors make the pattern of change much more variable than this expectation would suggest.

The first factor is that the long-term historical relationship of the doctor to the state does not always fit a picture of growing control over the profession. Germany is the most important illustration of this point. If we compare German doctors today with German doctors under Nazism from 1933 to 1945, the profession's independence now is immeasurably greater. And if we take a more recent time scale, the pattern is complex. The state has intervened more in the era of worries over costs. But to set against this we should note the transformation of the role of doctors in the previous (East) German Democratic Republic. Since re-unification, a system involving tight government control over a badly paid, low-status medical profession is being replaced by the pattern in the former 'West' Germany, where doctors enjoy high rewards and substantial independence. The example shows us that the history of individual countries must be borne in mind in examining the changing relationship of doctors to states.

A second factor causing variability in the changing relations of doctors and states is that, while everywhere the pressure to contain costs is intense, states do not always share the same interests, or need to use the same strategies, in trying to curb spending. The most direct reason for this is that states do not pick up the bill for health care to the same degree, nor do similar state institutions carry the costs in different countries. In the UK, most of health care is paid for by public spending raised through general taxation, and the chief paymaster and allocator of resources is national government. In Germany, the national, federal government in Bonn bears only a small proportion of total spending. The biggest share is split between a large number of health insurance funds operating, in practice, in varying degrees of independence from government institutions. In the USA, government contributes a minority share – though a very large minority, about 40 per cent – to the total cost of health care. It is part of a larger coalition of payers, encompassing employers, insurance companies and private patients. This is not to imply that, where the state does not directly pay, it is indifferent to those costs created by doctors. But it does indicate that, because states occupy different positions in health-care budgeting, their strategies will differ, and their relations with the medical profession will differ.

A third and final source of variability has recurred throughout this book. It concerns what, in summary, we can call the capacities of states. Even where a state wishes to exercise more control over the medical profession, it cannot always do so. The central institutions of the state in Germany, for instance, have been unable to control the entry of doctors to the profession, because responsibility for medical education is so dispersed in the governmental structure (it is largely the responsibility of the Länder). If anything, control has declined – the passing of the previous German Democratic Republic also abolished a system where the state in East Germany tightly regulated entry to medical schools.

More generally, all states suffer in varying degrees from an 'implementation gap' in their dealings with doctors: they can lay policies down, but carrying them out requires much larger amounts of resources and determination. That is why, in the UK case, it is still not clear how the formally tight controls introduced in the reforms of 1989–91 and will in practice constrain doctors. Equally, in the USA, it remains unclear whether the new Medicare fee schedules will be fully implemented and will impinge significantly on physician autonomy.

The argument of this book can be summed up in a few words: nations make a difference. We cannot simply offer generalizations about the power and role of the medical profession as if doctors were everywhere organized in the same way, and regulated in the same fashion. The work of doctors – how they are trained, employed and paid – is inexplicable without reference to the national setting in which medical work is done. History, political institutions, assumptions about the role and significance of medicine itself all reflect distinct national experiences.

Although nations make a difference, there is no single 'national character' at work in the regulation of doctors: the British are not uniformly attached to self-regulation, the Americans to regulation by the law. But the pattern that exists in each country is inexplicable without reference to the institutions, history and culture of that country. Of course national setting is not the only factor that matters. Another recurrent theme of this book has been the things that doctors have in common. Much of the scientific heritage of modern medicine is common to all advanced industrial societies, and thus many treatment practices are also common. We have also emphasized that many of the economic pressures on doctors, especially in recent years, have been similar in different countries. These common influences and pressures are, however, mediated through distinctive national institutions – and thus of necessity have different impacts on the medical professions of different nations. Thus, the final outcome of the regulatory process among physicians is the result of a complex interaction between national uniqueness and shared influences.

FUTHER READING

The general thesis that doctors are in decline has been proposed, in rather different forms, by Starr (1982); by Starr and Immergut (1987); by McKinlay and Arches

(1985) and by McKinlay and Stoeckle (1988). It has been denied by Elston (1991) and is treated sceptically by Döhler (1989). The idea that doctors are central to the wider (non-medical) functioning of welfare states is explored in Stone (1984). The 'power of doctors' debate is given a historical perspective by De Swaan (1989). Some of the many protagonists debate the issues in a valuable special issue of the *Milbank Quarterly*, Supplement 2 (1988). For specific reading on the countries considered here, and on the four regulatory issues (entry, competition, market structures, pay) see the Further Reading at the end of preceding chapters.

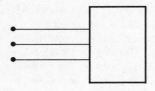

REFERENCES

Aaron, H.J. and Schwartz, W.B. (1984) *The Painful Prescription: Rationing Hospital Care*, Washington DC: Brookings Institution.

Alber, J. (1989) *Der Sozialstaat in der Bundesrepublik 1950–83*, Frankfurt: Campus.

Alber, J. (1991) 'The West German health care system in comparative perspective', in E. Kolinsky (ed.) *The Federal Republic of Germany: The End of an Era*, New York: Berg.

Alford, R.R. (1975) *Health Care Politics*, Chicago: University of Chicago Press.

Allsop, J. (1984) *Health Policy and the National Health Service*, London: Longman.

Altenstetter, C. (1989) 'Hospital planners and medical professionals in the Federal Republic of Germany', in G. Freddi and J. Björkman (eds) *Controlling Medical Professionals*, London: Sage.

Baggott, R. (1989) 'Regulatory reform in Britain: the changing face of self-regulation', *Public Administration*, 67(4), 435–54.

Baier, H. (1988) *Ehrlichkeit in Sozialstaat: Gesundheit zwischen Medizin und Manipulation*, Osnabrück: Fromm.

Bauch, J. (1982) 'Zwischen Gesinnungsethik und Verbandszwang: Ärtzverbände als Korrektiv der soziologischen Organisationstheorie', *Soziale Welt*, 33(2), 221–35.

Baumol, W.J. (1988) 'Containing medical costs: why price controls won't work', *Public Interest*, 93, 37–53.

Björkman, J. (1989) 'Politicizing medicine and medical politics: physician power in the United States', in G. Freddi and J. Björkman (eds) *Controlling Medical Professionals*, London: Sage.

Blank, R.H. (1988) *Rationing Medicine*, New York: Columbia University Press.

Breyer, F., Paffrath, D., Preuss, W. and Schmidt, R. (1987) *Die Krankenhauskosten-funktion*, Bonn: AOK Verlag.

Butterfass, E. (1986) 'Freie Ärtzverbände – Gewerkschaften oder Berufsverbände', *Medizin, Mensch und Gessellschaft*, 11, 30–4.

Campion, F. (1984) *The American Medical Association and United States Health Policy since 1940*, Chicago: Chicago Review Press.

Carr-Saunders, A.M. and Wilson, P.A. (1933) *The Professions*, Oxford: Oxford University Press.

Cohen, H.S. (1980) 'On professional power and conflict of interest: state licensing boards on trial', *Journal of Health Politics, Policy and Law*, 5(2), 291–308.

Colombotos, J. and Kirchner, C. (1986) *Physicians and Social Change*, Oxford: Oxford University Press.

Cyffka, J. (1988) 'Zur Belastung von Krankenkassen durch die Folgen der Arbeitslosigkeit', *Die Ortskrankenkassen* (July 1988), 400–4.

Day, P. and Klein, R. (1991) 'Britain's health care experiment', *Health Affairs*, 10(3), 39–59.

Department of Health (1990) *Consultants' Distinction Awards*, London: Department of Health (UK).

Deppe, H.-U. (1987a) *Krankheit ist ohne Politik nicht heilbar*, Frankfurt: Suhrkamf.

Deppe, H.-U (1987b) 'Zulassungssperre: Ärtze in den Fesseln der Standespolitik', in H.-U. Deppe, H. Friedrich and R. Müllaer (eds) *Medizin und Gessellschaft*, Frankfurt: Campus.

De Swaan, A. (1989) 'The reluctant imperialism of the medical profession', *Social Science and Medicine*, 28(11), 1165–70.

Deutsche Bundesbank (1991) 'Recent trends in the finances of the statutory health insurance institutions', *Monthly Report* (January), 25–36.

Döhler, M. (1989) 'Physicians' professional autonomy in the welfare state: endangered or preserved?', in G. Freddi, and J. Björkman *Controlling Medical Professionals*, London: Sage.

Döhler, M. (1991) 'Policy networks, opportunity structures and neo-conservative reform strategies in health policy', in B. Marin and R. Mayntz, (eds) *Policy Networks: Empirical Evidence and Theoretical Considerations*, Frankfurt: Campus.

Elston, M. (1991) 'The politics of professional power: medicine in a changing health service', in J. Gabe, M. Calnan and M. Bury (eds) *The Sociology of the Health Service*, London: Routledge.

Enthoven, A.C. (1991) 'Internal market reform of the British health service', *Health Affairs*, 10(3), 60–70.

Ermann, D. (1988) 'Hospital Utilization Review: past experience, future directions', *Journal of Health Politics, Policy and Law*, 13(4), 683–704.

Field, M.J. and Gray, B.H. (1989) 'Should we regulate "utilisation management"?', *Health Affairs*, 8(4), 103–12.

Folland, S.T. (1985) 'The effects of health care advertising', *Journal of Health Politics, Policy and Law*, 10(2), 329–45.

Fox, D.M. (1987) *Health Policies, Health Politics: The British and American Experience, 1911–1965*, Princeton, NJ: Princeton University Press.

Freddi, G. (1989) 'Problems of organizational rationality in health systems: political controls and policy options', in G. Freddi and J. Björkman (eds) *Controlling Medical Professionals*, London: Sage.

Freddi, G. and Björkman, J.W. (eds) (1989) *Controlling Medical Professionals: The Comparative Politics of Health Governance*, London: Sage.

Freidson, E. (1970) *Profession of Medicine: A Study of the Sociology of Applied Knowledge*, New York: Dodd Mead.

Gaumer, G.L. (1984) 'Regulating health professionals: a review of the empirical literature', *Milbank Quarterly*, 62(3), 380–416.

Ginsburg, P.B., LeRoy, L.B. and Hammons, G.T. (1990) 'Medicare physician payment reform', *Health Affairs*, 9(1), 178–88.

Gockenjaan, G. (1987) 'Nicht länger Lohnsklaven und Pfenningskulis? Zur Entwicklung der niedergelassenen Ärzte', in H. Deppe, H. Friedrich and R. Müller (eds) *Medizin und Gessellschaft*, Frankfurt: Campus.

Godt, P.J. (1987) 'Confrontation, consent and corporatism: state strategies and the medical profession in France, Great Britain and West Germany', *Journal of Health Politics, Policy and Law*, 12(3), 459–80.

Gold, M. and Hodges, D. (1989) 'Health Maintenance Organisations in 1988', *Health Affairs* 8(4), 125–38.

Gould, D. (1985) *The Black and White Medicine Show*, London: Hamish Hamilton.

Gray, B.H. (ed.) (1983) *The New Health Care for Profit: Doctors and Hospitals in a Competitive Environment*, Washington DC: National Academy Press.

Gross, S.J. (1984) *Of Foxes and Hen Houses: Licensing and the Health Professions*, Westport, Conn: Quorum Books.

Grumbach, K. and Bodenheimer, T. (1990) 'Reins or fences: a physician's view of cost containment', *Health Affairs* 9(4), 120–6.

Ham, C. (1992) *Health Policy in Britain*, 3rd edn, London: Macmillan.

Ham, C., Robinson, R. and Benzeval, M. (1990) *Health check: Health Care Reforms in an International Context*, London: King's Fund Institute.

Harrison, S., Hunter, D.J. and Pollitt, C. (1990) *The Dynamics of British Health Policy*, London: Unwin Hyman.

Haug, M.R. (1976) 'The erosion of professional authority: a cross-cultural inquiry in the case of the physician', *Milbank Quarterly*, 54(1), 83–106.

Haug, M.R. (1988) 'A re-examination of the hypothesis of physician deprofessionalization', *Milbank Quarterly*, 66(2), 48–56.

Havighurst, C.C., Helms, R.B., Bladen, C. and Pauly, M.V. (1989) *American Health Care – what are the lessons for Britain?*, London: Institute of Economic Affairs Health Unit.

Heidenheimer, A.J. (1973) 'The politics of public education, health and welfare in the USA and Western Europe: how growth and reform potentials have differed', *British Journal of Political Science*, 3(3), 315–40.

Heidenheimer, A.J. (1980) 'Organised medicine and physician specialization in Scandinavia and West Germany', *West European Politics*, 3(3), 373–87.

Heidenheimer, A.J., Heclo, H. and Teich Adams, C. (1990) *Comparative Public Policy*, 3rd edn, New York: St Martin's Press.

Henke, K.D. (1986) 'A concerted approach to health care financing in the Federal Republic of Germany', *Health Policy* 6(3), 341–51.

Henke, K.D. (1991) 'Fiscal problems of German unity – the case of health care', *Staatswissesnschaft und Staatspraxis*, (2), 170–9.

Hiatt, H. (1987) *America's Health in the Balance: Choice or Change?*, New York: Harper and Row.

Hurst, J. (1991) 'Reform of health care in Germany', *Health Care Financing Review*, 12(3), 73–85.

Iglehart, J.K. (1991a) 'Germany's health care system, Part 1', *New England Journal of Medicine*, 324, 503–8.

Iglehart, J.K. (1991b) 'Germany's health care system, Part 2', *New England Journal of Medicine*, 324, 1750–6.

Inlander, C.B., Levin, L.S., and Weiner, E. (1988) *Medicine on Trial: The Appalling Story of Ineptitude, Malfeasance, Neglect and Arrogance*, Englewood Cliffs, NJ: Prentice Hall.

JAMA (1988a) 'Report on the accreditation process', *Journal of the American Medical Association*, 259, 1058–9.

JAMA (1988b) 'Report on medical licensure', *Journal of the American Medical Association*, 259, 1994–2001.

JAMA (1988c) 'Permanent injunction order against AMA', *Journal of the American Medical Association*, 259, 81–2.

Jennings, B. (1987) 'The professions: public interest and common good', *Hastings Center Report*, 17(1), Supplement, 3–10.

Johnson, T. (1972) *Professions and Power*, London: Macmillan.

Karcher, H. (1990) 'Merging German health care systems', *British Medical Journal*, 7 April, 894.

Katzenstein, P. (1987) *Policy and Politics in West Germany: The Growth of a Semi-Sovereign State*, Philadelphia: Temple University Press.

Klein, R. (1981) 'Reflections on the American health care condition', *Journal of Health Politics, Policy and Law*, 6(2), 188–204.

Klein, R. (1989) *The Politics of the NHS*, 2nd edn, London: Longman.

Larkin, G. (1983) *Occupational Monopoly and Modern Medicine*, London: Tavistock.

Levin, A. (ed.) (1980) *Regulating health care: the struggle for control*, New York: Academy of Political Science.

Lubecki, P. (1987) 'Zulassungsbeschränkungen für Kassenärzte', *Die Ortskrankenkassen* (1 April), 194–208.

Lubecki, P. (1989) 'Kriterion für Zulassengsperren', *Die Ortskrankenkassen* (15 March), 194–6.

Ludmerer, K. (1985) *Learning to Heal: The Development of American Medical Education*, New York: Basic Books.

McKeown, T. (1980) *The Role of Medicine: Dream, Mirage or Nemesis?*, 2nd edn, Oxford: Blackwell.

McKinlay, J. and Arches, J. (1985) 'Towards the proletarianization of physicians', *International Journal of Health Services*, 15(2), 161–95.

McKinlay, J.B. and Stoeckle, J.D. (1988) 'Corporatization and the social transformation of doctoring', *International Journal of Health Services*, 18(2), 191–205.

Mark, S. (1986) *Die Stenerung ambulanter medizinischer Leistungen im Gesundkeitssystem*, Cologne: Centaurus.

Marmor, T.R. and Thomas, D. (1972) 'Doctors, politics and pay disputes: "pressure group politics" revisited', *British Journal of Political Science*, 2(4), 421–42.

Mechanic, D. (1985) 'Physicians and patients in transition', *Hastings Center Report*, 15(6), 9–12.

Milbank Quarterly (1988) special issue on 'The changing character of the medical profession', 66, Supplement 2.

Moran, M. (1990) *Distributional struggles in the German health care system*, European Policy Research Unit, University of Manchester.

Murswieck, A. (1985) 'Health policy making', in K. von Beyme and M. Schmidt (eds) *Policy and Politics in the Federal Republic of Germany*, Aldershot: Dartmouth.

OECD (1985) *Measuring Health Care 1960–83*, Paris: OECD.

OECD (1987) *Financing and Delivering Health Care*, Paris: OECD.

OECD (1990) *Health Care Systems in Transition*, Paris, OECD.

Oldiges, F. (1988) 'Verfassungsfragen der Zulassung als Kassenarzt', *Die Ortskrankenkassen* (15 June), 357–62.

Oppl, H. and von Kordoff, E. (1990) 'The National Health Care System in the welfare state', *Social Science and Medicine*, 31(1), 43–50.

Pick, P. and Plein, J. (1989) 'Betriebskrankenkassen: Risikoselektion versus Solidarprinzip', *Die Ortskrankenkassen* (1 June), 297–303.

Pollitt, C. (1990) 'Doing business in the temple? Managers and quality assurance in the public services', *Public Administration*, 68(4), 435–52.

Raffel, M.W. and Raffel, N.K. (1989) *The United States Health System: Origins and Functions*, 3rd edn, New York: John Wiley.

Richman, J. (1987) *Medicine and Health*, London: Longman.

Rodwin, V.G. (1989) 'Physician payment reform: lessons from abroad', *Health Affairs*, 8(4), 76–83.

Rosenberg, P. (1986) 'The origin and development of compulsory insurance in Germany', in D.W. Light and A. Schuller (eds) *Political Values and Health Care: the German Experience*, Cambridge, Mass.: MIT Press.

Schardt, T. and Wendt, G. (1987) 'Ärzteschwemme', in H. Deppe, H. Friedrich and R. Müller (eds) *Medizin und Gessellschaft*, Frankfurt: Campus.

Schieber, G.J., Poullier, J.-P. and Greenwald, L.M. (1991) 'Health care systems in twenty-four countries', *Health Affairs*, 10(3), 22–38.

Schneider, M. (1991) 'Health care cost containment in the Federal Republic of Germany', *Health Care Financing Review*, 12(3), 87–101.

Scholmer, J. (1984) *Das Geschäft mit der Krankheit*, Cologne: Kiepeneuer and Witsch.

Schramm, C.J. (ed.) (1987) *Health Care and its Costs*, New York: Norton.

Schwartz, W.B. and Mendelson, D.N. (1989) 'The role of physician-owned insurance companies in the detection and deterrence of negligence', *Journal of the American Medical Association*, 262, 1342–6.

Stacey, M. (1989) 'The General Medical Council and professional accountability', *Public Policy and Administration*, 4(1), 12–27.

Starr, P. (1982) *The Social Transformation of American Medicine*, New York: Basic Books.

Starr, P. and Immergut, E. (1987) 'Health care and the boundaries of politics', in C. Maier (ed.) *Changing Boundaries of the Political*, Cambridge: Cambridge University Press.

Stone, D. (1977) 'Professionalism and accountability: controlling health services in the United States and West Germany', *Journal of Health Politics, Policy and Law*, 2(1), 32–47.

Stone, D. (1980a) 'The problem of monopoly power in federal health policy', *Milbank Quarterly*, 58(1), 50–3.

Stone, D. (1980b) *The Limits of Professional Power: National Health Care in the Federal Republic of Germany*, Chicago: University of Chicago Press.

Stone, D. (1984) *The Disabled State*, London: Macmillan.

Strong, P. and Robinson, J. (1990) *The NHS – Under New Management*, Milton Keynes: Open University Press.

Tennstedt, F. (1977) *Soziale Selbsterverwaltung: Geschichte der Selbsterverwaltung in der Krankenversicherung*, Cologne: Verlag der Ortskrankenkassen.

Van den Busche, H. (1990) 'The history and future of physician manpower development in the Federal Republic of Germany', *Health Policy*, 15, 215–31.

Vogel, D. (1986) *National Styles of Regulation*, Ithaca, NY: Cornell University Press.

Von Ferber, C. (1989) 'Strukturreform oder Weiterentwicklung des gegliederten Sozialleistungsystems der Bundesrepublik?', in G. Löschen, W.C. Cockerham and G. Kunz (eds) *Gesundheit und Krankheit in der BRD and den USA*, Munich: Oldenburg Verlag.

Walsh, D.C. (1987) *Corporate Physicians: Between Medicine and Management*, New Haven, Conn.: Yale University Press.

Webber, D. (1988) 'Krankheit, Geld und Politik: Zur Geschichte der Gesundheitsreformen in Deutschland', *Leviathan*, 16(2), 156–203.

Webber, D. (1989) 'Zur Geschichte der Gesundheitsreformen in Deutschland – II, Norbert Blüms Gesundheitsreform und die Lobby', *Leviathan*, 17, 262–300.

Webber, D. (1991) 'Health policy and the Christian–Liberal coalition in West Germany: the conflicts over the Health Insurance Reform, 1987–8', in C. Altenstetter and S.C. Haywood (eds) *Comparative Health Policy and the New Right*, London: Macmillan.

Weiner, J.P. (1989) 'Forecasting physician supply: recent developments', *Health Affairs*, 8(4), 173–9.

Wendt, G. (1985) 'Disparitäten in der ambulanten ärztlichen Versorgung' in H. Deppe, U. Gerhardt and P. Novak (eds) *Medizinische Soziologie*, Frankfurt: Campus.

Wilding, P. (1982) *Professional Power and Social Welfare*, London: Routledge.

Wilsford, D. (1991) *Doctors and the State: The Politics of Health Care in France and the United States*, Durham, NC: Duke University Press.

Wood, B. (1991) 'The non-achievement of cost containment in American health care: explanations, and lessons for Britain', *Public Policy and Administration*, 6(3), 22–39.

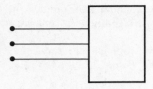

INDEX